Veröffentlichungen aus der
Geomedizinischen Forschungsstelle
(Leiter: Professor Dr. Dr. h.c. mult. G. Schettler)
der Heidelberger Akademie der Wissenschaften

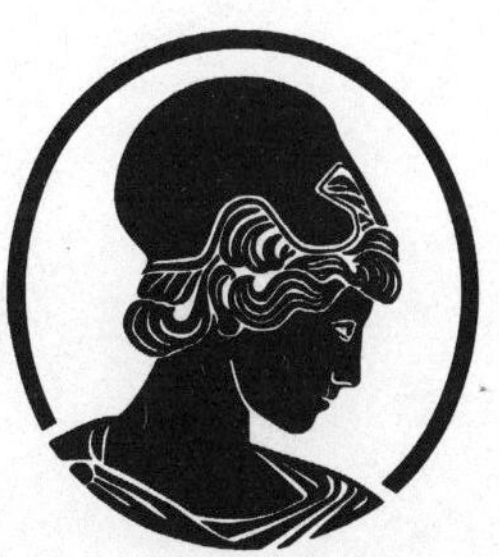

Supplement zu den Sitzungsberichten der
Mathematisch-naturwissenschaftlichen Klasse
Jahrgang 1992

W. Morgenstern E. Chigan R. Prokhorskas
M. Rusnak G. Schettler (Eds.)

Models of Noncommunicable Diseases

Health Status and Health Service Requirements

With 23 Figures and 36 Tables

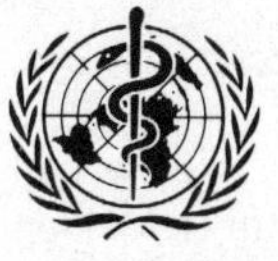

Published in collaboration with the
World Health Organization

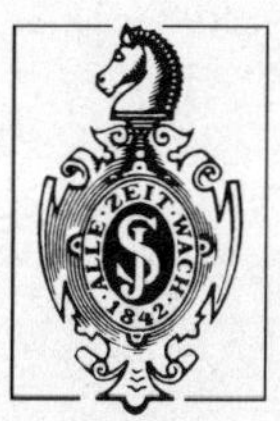

Springer-Verlag
Berlin Heidelberg New York
London Paris Tokyo
Hong Kong Barcelona
Budapest

Dipl.- Math. Wolfgang Morgenstern
Geomedical Research Unit
Heidelberg Academy for the Humanities and Sciences
Karlstraße 4, W-6900 Heidelberg, FRG

Dr. Evgueni Chigan
Headquarters, World Health Organization
CH-1211 Geneva 27, Switzerland

Dr. Rimidius Prokhorskas
Regional Office for Europe, World Health Organization
Scherfigsvej 8, DK-2100 Copenhagen, Denmark

Dr. Martin Rusnak
Medical Informatics Research Institute
Jedlova 6, 83308 Bratislava, Czechoslovakia

Prof. Dr. Dr. h.c. mult. Gotthard Schettler
Geomedical Research Unit
Heidelberg Academy for the Humanities and Sciences
Karlstraße 4, W-6900 Heidelberg, FRG

The views expressed in this book do not necessarily represent the decisions or the stated policy of the World Health Organization

---

ISBN 3-540-55217-0 Springer-Verlag Berlin Heidelberg New York
ISBN 0-387-55217-0 Springer-Verlag New York Berlin Heidelberg

Printed in Germany

Typesetting: Camera ready by author

25/3140-543210 - Printed on acid-free paper

Contents

List of Contributors

Andel, M., Dr.
IInd Clinic of Internal Medicine
Královské Vinohrady Teaching Hospital
Srobárova 50, 100 34 Prague 2, Czechoslovakia

Aromaa, A., Dr
Research Institute for Social Security
Social Insurance Institution
P. O. Box 78, 00381 Helsinki, Finland

Barendregt, J. J. M., Dr.
Department of Public Health and Social Medicine
Erasmus University
P. B. 1738, 3000 DR Rotterdam, The Netherlands

Bonneux, L., Dr.
Department of Public Health and Social Medicine
Erasmus University
P. B. 1738, 3000 DR Rotterdam, The Netherlands

Capocaccia, R., Dr.
Laboratory of Epidemiology and Biostatistics
Istituto Superiore di Sanitá
Viale Regina Elena 299, 00161 Rome, Italy

Chigan, E. N., Dr.
Headquarters, World Health Organization
1211 Geneva 27, Switzerland

Cider, B.
Research Institute of Medical Informatics
Jedlova 6, 833 08 Bratislava, Czechoslovakia

Gunning-Schepers, L. J., Prof. Dr.
Department of Public Health and Social Medicine
University of Amsterdam
Meibergdreef 15, 1105 AZ Amsterdam, The Netherlands

Habbema, J. D. F., Dr.
Department of Public Health and Social Medicine
Erasmus University
P. B. 1738, 3000 DR Rotterdam, The Netherlands

Hauser, F., Ing.
Institute of Social Medicine
and Health Services Organization
Palackého nám. 4, 128 00 Prague, Czechoslovakia

Heliövaara, M., Dr.
Research Institute for Social Security
Social Insurance Institution
P. O. Box 78, 00381 Helsinki, Finland

van Hout, B. A., Dr.
Institute for Medical Technology Assessment
Erasmus University, Medical Faculty
P. O. Box 1738, 3000 DR Rotterdam, The Netherlands

Knekt, P., Dr.
Research Institute for Social Security
Social Insurance Institution
P. O. Box 78, 00381 Helsinki, Finland

Kotva, M., Ing.
PTT Research Institute
Hvoždanská 3, 149 50 Prague 4, Czechoslovakia

van der Maas, P. J., Dr.
Department of Public Health and Social Medicine
Erasmus University
P. B. 1738, 3000 DR Rotterdam, The Netherlands

Manton, K. G., Prof. Dr.
Center for Demographic Studies
Duke University
2117 Campus Drive, Durham, NC 27706, U. S. A.

Michalski, A. I., Dr.
Institute of Control Sciences, Academy of Sciences
Profsoyuznaya 65, 117806 GSP - 7. Moscow, Russia

Morgenstern, W., Dipl. Math.
Geomedical Research Unit
Heidelberg Academy for the Humanities and Sciences
Karlstraße 4, 6900 Heidelberg, Germany

McPherson, K., Prof. Dr.
Health Promotion Sciences Unit
Department of Public Health and Policy
London School of Hygiene and Tropical Medicine
Ceppel Street, London VC1 E7 HT, United Kingdom

Prokhorskas, R., Dr.
Unit of Epidemiology, Statistics and Research
Regional Office for Europe, World Health Organization
Scherfigsvej 8, 2100 Copenhagen Ø, Denmark

Reunanen, A., Dr.
Research Institute for Social Security
Social Insurance Institution
P. O. Box 78, 00381 Helsinki, Finland

Rissanen, A., Dr.
Research Institute for Social Security
Social Insurance Institution
P. O. Box 78, 00381 Helsinki, Finland

Rusnak, M., Dr.
Research Institute of Medical Informatics
Jedlova 6, 833 08 Bratislava, Czechoslovakia

Scherbov, S., Dr.
Population Research Centre
University of Groningen, Faculty of Spatial Sciences
P. O. B. 800, 9700 AV Groningen, The Netherlands

Stallard, E., Dr.
Center for Demographic Studies, Duke University
2117 Campus Drive, Durham, NC 27706, U. S. A.

Taket, A. R., Dr.
Dept. of Geography, Queen Mary and Westfield College
University of London
Mile End Road, London E1 4NS, United Kingdom

Woodbury, M. A., Prof. Dr.
Center for Demographic Studies, Duke University
2117 Campus Drive, Durham, NC 27706, U. S. A.

Yashin, A. I., Dr.
Institute of Control Sciences, Academy of Sciences
Profsoyuznaya 65, 117806 GSP - 7. Moscow, Russia

Introduction

E. N. Chigan

The set of sixteen papers published here under the title: *Models of Noncommunicable Diseases: Health Status and Health Service Requirements* have been selected from a series of reports presented at two recent workshops held under the auspices of the World Health Organization and respectively hosted by the Heidelberg Academy for the Humanities and Sciences and the Medical Bionics Research Institute, Bratislava, Czechoslovakia.

These workshops, organized by the Division of Noncommunicable Diseases and Health Technology at WHO Headquarters, and by the European Regional Office of WHO, are the most recent of a series of workshops held approximately every two years since 1984 as part of a WHO Programme in the Modelling of Noncommunicable Diseases.

The main aim of the WHO Programme is to ensure that available or potentially available epidemiological data on noncommunicable diseases are appropriately applied to health planning processes aimed at the reduction of incidence, prevalence, disability and mortality due to these diseases. Those disease prevention and control programmes in noncommunicable disease that deal with changing life styles or behavior at the community level or with changes in other external risk factors, are seen as situations where it is necessary to evaluate the impact of various health intervention programmes to prioritize the composition of the components of a given strategy in a given country.

The modelling effort explicitly entails measuring the basic components of risk factor change, their impact on multiple disease end points, the costs of the intervention and the social and economic consequences of the impact, including demand for health services. The standard forms of epidemiological data presentation on risk factor impacts such as relative risk and population attributable risks, or multiple logistic equation coefficients are not usually useful impact measures for population prevention programmes since they do not directly relate the demographic and risk factor interrelationships which determine impact in these populations.

To be useful for planning purposes, models need the following characteristics:

- a time dimension over which risk factors may develop, e.g. with age, or by period effects, with latent periods before risk factors impact morbidity and mortality, and with lag times during which risk factor changes are translated into mortality reduction;

- a multifactorial representation of risk factors and diseases where one risk factor may influence several diseases, and one disease may be influenced by several risk factors;
- a demographic basis by which population changes occurring over the forecasting period can be considered;
- a set of actuarial measures by which social and economic impacts can be incorporated into the planning process. For mortality, this involves the use of multiple decrement life table output parameters which can be related to the population structure of specific countries or regions;
- a set of health service needs measures based upon the demographic and epidemiologic status of the population as expressed by morbidity, disability and mortality incidences and prevalences for various age, sex, socio-economic and geographically distributed population groups.

These five points are addressed by the sixteen papers found in this issue. The papers by Kotva, and Bonneux and Barendregt deal with conceptual issues relating to the validity and verifiability of models. Both point out problems of dealing with complex but seldom verifiable sets of assumptions necessary to incorporate all the characteristics appropriate for noncommunicable disease models as opposed to a simpler model specification which better utilizes available data, but which do not necessarily reproduce the *real world* situation.

Rusnak gives an overview of current trends in the modelling of noncommunicable diseases and their effects on the health care system. This review is done taking into account the potential users of the model, the *user-friendliness* of the model, and the availability of data for appropriate use of the model in a specific planning situation.

Papers by Capocaccia and by Michalski and Yashin deal with the problems of estimating disease morbidity from disease mortality data in those situations where incidence and prevalence data are not available for a chronic disease. These papers use explicit assumptions on unobserved relationships between morbidity and mortality in cancers to overcome lack of morbidity data.

Gunning-Schepers, Barendregt and van der Maas describe a model incorporating latent and lag periods for risk factor changes and the demographic structure of the population when predicting chronic disease mortality. The paper by McPherson also stresses the need to consider the delayed effects of exposure to a risk factor (oral contraceptive) when estimating risk of disease (breast cancer).

The reports of Hauser and Andel, and of Rusnak, Scherbov and Cider demonstrate the use of multi-state transition models to produce projections for morbidity and mortality from specific diseases. Both reports stress the need to include demographic structure of the population explicitly in the model.

Heliövaara et al., using a simpler predictive model, show how risk factors thought to be specific for cardiovascular mortality may also predict work disability but through quite different demographic and disease patterns.

Manton, Stallard and Woodbury, and Michalski both use a more mathematically complex stochastic process model to deal with the problems of multidimensional measures of health status and competing risks in heterogeneous populations.

Prokhorskas suggests the use of a generalized relative risk function which better represents the way in which mortality and morbidity risks change with changing levels of risk factors. He illustrates this with data pooled from several studies.

In a review paper, Taket explores the current situation in modelling health services resource allocation and their potential linkages to health status measures and to other key factors in the health system.

As an example of modelling in technology assessment, van Hout and Habbema present a stochastic compartment model to cost and effects (quality of life) in a heart transplant programme. While the heart transplant example might seem far removed from primary prevention programmes, the same cost-effectiveness modelling techniques obviously apply to less *high-tech* interventions.

All of the foregoing papers emphasize the need for appropriate, reliable and sufficient data for developing, calibrating and implementing models at national and sub-national levels. Generally speaking, the more biologically realistic the model, the more demanding are its needs for extensive data sets. Morgenstern addresses this issue by demonstrating how local risk factor data may provide reasonable estimates of national coronary heart disease mortality rates.

In addition to need for appropriate data bases to use in model development and implementation, two other issues appear in several papers:

- the need to identify and sensitize potential users of models among health managers and health planners;
- the need to incorporate disease modelling into the curriculum of courses dealing with epidemiological methods and health planning.

In addition to further development and extension of existing disease process models and their linkage to delivery of health services, these last three concerns need to be added to the agenda for future health modelling efforts.

Some Conceptual Problems in the Simulation of Epidemiological Processes

M. Kotva

Introduction

The simulation of epidemiological processes involves a number of more or less specific conceptual problems. As a result, the simulation of systems, a specific form of the process of cognition, has up to now rarely been used in this field. Particular attention should be paid to the *data-model* relationship, and especially to the problems of testing the validity of a simulation model (i.e., of verifying that a simulation model conforms to objective reality).

The Data - Model Relationship

There are a number of scientific disciplines which, owing to the complexity of the subject being studied, the limited possibilities of experimentation (as well as of observation and measurement), and an inadequate social demand, have not yet attained a very high level of cognition. It is mainly in these disciplines that one finds a biased understanding of the *data - model* relationship. The models are viewed exclusively as the interpretation of observed data concerning the object being studied. This conception prevails in epidemiology. It represents the main obstacle to a wider use of systems simulation in this discipline, because it is in direct contradiction with the nature of simulation as a specific form of the process of cognition [1].

We do not, of course, deny the important role of observed data in the process of systems simulation. A simulation model is created on the basis of our idea of the investigated system and its *motion* (how it reacts on stimuli from outside, the changes in its structure, quality, etc.). This idea is derived through a deductive process from hitherto verified scientific explanations and theories, as well as through an inductive process from hitherto observed data. However an inductive process, even if used correctly, may lead to false conclusions. Therefore, in testing *correctness* of a simulation model (whether it conforms to our idea), we should verify it, not only by comparing the *motion* of the simulation model with the results of thought experiments based on our idea (these being over-simplified in the case of complex problems), but also by seeing whether the model accurately interprets the data from which this idea has been derived. It is, of course, necessary to verify whether the *motion* of the simulation model agrees with our existing knowledge. Hence, the model should be understood as a representation of our knowledge and hypotheses about the object under study, rather than a mere tool for interpreting hitherto observed data.

Verification that the simulation model *truthfully* interprets observed data thus represents the conclusion of *testing correctness of the simulation model.* It is the first, and only the first, step towards *testing validity of the simulation model*, in the sense of verifying that the model is adequate in relation to the real object. For other steps we must obtain new data, starting therein from the basic principle of the verification of scientific hypotheses. We must therefore ask ourselves: *What should (or should not) be observed if the hypothesis is true?.* The answer can be given by experiments with the simulation model, which thus replace the thought experiments. The specificity of the simulation of systems as a specific form of the process of cognition consists precisely of this replacement. We should then repeat the experiment carried out with the simulation model, with the simulated system under the same conditions. If the *truthfulness* of the conclusions drawn from the simulation experiment is confirmed in this way, this increases the probability (or our conviction) that the simulation model is valid, and consequently that the hypotheses represented by it are valid. The more surprising (or even contrary to *common sense*) are the conclusions drawn from the experiments, then the more likely is it that the model is valid. On the other hand, if the prediction or conclusions are shown to be invalid, this refutes the hypotheses, or at least weakens our conviction of their truthfulness [2].

It is the difficulty, or sheer impossibility, of testing validity of the model by experimenting on a real object which causes the above-mentioned understanding and using models only as the interpretation of observed data. For the time being, when simulating epidemiological processes related to noncommunicable diseases, it is usually impossible to advance further towards the verification of models. Let us therefore ask ourselves two basic questions:

- Are we justified in using unverified models in support of decision-making in health care management?
- Will it be possible to advance further in the verification of epidemiological models?

The Use of Unverified Epidemiological Simulation Models

Problems related to the applicability of unverified simulation models were vividly illustrated by the discussion reported in the second half of 1988, in the journal Science.

David Dickson's article about IIASA [3] provoked a letter from Saunders MacLane [4], which in turn brought disagreement from Harvey Brooks, Alan McDonald, and Nathan Keyfitz [5]. Regardless of IIASA and of Forrester's *Systems Dynamics*, the main point of contention is the question of how admissible is the use of unverified models in support of decision-making, in such sensitive areas of world development as ecology or energy. In our view, there is some truth on both sides. MacLane is indisputably correct when he protests against the use of unverified models. Brooks, McDonald, and especially Keyfitz are equally correct in asking what else could be done in the present state of knowledge, when verified models are not yet available, and while problems refuse to wait for models to be completed. Just this dilemma led the Czechoslovak Scientific and Technological Society, as long as 1977, to adopt an agreement on understanding the notion *simulation of systems*. In a narrower sense, this is understood as the method of experiments with a simulation model, but in a broader sense as a specific form of cognition process [1]. When, at the very beginning, a simulation model is applied to the investigation of a real object, it is always unverified (otherwise we could hardly speak of *investigation*), and one cannot be sure if it is correct.

After checking the model for correctness, which is nearly always possible, experiments can be carried out with it in order to make forecasts based on our ideas. However, these ideas may be partially or even completely wrong and, in the same way, the resulting forecasts may also be wrong. Although the outcome is the same whether we use a thought or simulation model, the use of the latter has the following advantages: first, a heuristic contribution to the completeness of our ideas, and coherence of all their aspects; second, the possibility of quantifying our ideas according to available data; and third, the ability to perform substantially more complex experiments than is possible with thought models. In any case, conclusions reached by means of a simulation model that has been checked for correctness but not for validity (i.e., by means of a model which has the character of a mere hypothesis) should be considered as hypothetical only.

It is, of course, necessary to verify hypotheses, even if this is only partially possible. Paradoxical as it may seem, the use of hypothetical simulation models for health care management represents a step towards their verification, on condition that we understand and use them in this way. This leads us to the second question which we have raised.

Possibilities of Testing the Validity of Epidemiological Simulation Models

One can regard an epidemiological forecast based on experiments with hypothetical simulation model also as a statement *what should be observed if the hypothesis (on which this model is based) is true?* Hence, the verification of such a forecast thus strengthens our convictions that the hypothesis is true. In a negative case, assumptions made about the impact of external factors need to be verified, since the accuracy of a forecast depends on them as well as on the hypothesis. When these assumptions proved to be wrong, only the repetition of simulation experiments under conditions corresponding to the now already known real situation can definitively strengthen or weaken our conviction about the truthfulness of the used hypothesis.

This way of verifying the simulation models of epidemiological processes is very lengthy, partly because it is dependent on the native rather than experimental conditions. Hence, one cannot verify forecasts made by means of simulation model which are *surprising* or *contrary to common sense* which can speed up the process of verification. There is, however, another way which could bring results more quickly, but which requires a fundamental change in the method of gathering epidemiological data.

At present, the gathering of epidemiological data represents a complex problem. Data provided by existing statistical information systems in health care are limited and not always reliable, because they are based on episodes and not on real people. More valuable data, in this respect, are available from various registers of diseases, of high-risk groups, of deaths, etc. However such registers, as well as various surveys, selective investigations, or longitudinal studies, are expensive and time-consuming, especially in view of their single-purpose use and narrow, specialized orientation. Despite the advent of modern computer technology, the traditional statistical-descriptive approach still survives. Various centralized registers are developed as data banks fed by routine reports and periodic censuses and surveys. The common shortcoming of virtually all the above-mentioned sources of epidemiological data is their prevailing orientation towards illness or patients, rather than towards health and the population as a whole, including healthy individuals.

There exists one way out of this situation. The documentation produced by *first contact physicians* contains an inexhaustible, but virtually inaccessible, amount of information needed for epidemiological studies. If physicians could save this information on personal computers, and if a national, hierarchically structured health care information system could be developed, then not only would such data contribute to the immediate practice and management of health care, but undreamed-of possibilities would emerge for socio-medical and epidemiological research. In such a situation, it would be inexcusable to continue applying only the traditional approaches to epidemiological studies. One of the most important new approaches would consist of the simulation of epidemiological processes whose extensive use would be made possible by the availability of necessary data.

This leads us back to the *data-model* relationship. While today we are forced to subordinate the creation of models, if we undertake it at all, to the imperative of data accessibility, the above-mentioned information system would offer an almost unlimited supply of data for creating hypotheses and, subsequently, for creating simulation models and testing their validity. An obvious prerequisite is that these uses and at the same time *roofing* for the information system be foreseen from the very outset. Simulation models could and should play a dual role. On the one hand, they could help to decide which data should be available in the information system, in addition to those required for immediate medical practice. This presupposes that we begin at once to create epidemiological (and other) simulation models, irrespective of the present lack of inaccessible data which are necessary for the quantification of their parameters, as well as for testing their validity. The simulation models, on the other hand, should be thought of as a *roofing* element of the whole information system, for applications which will serve the needs of health care decision-making.

Health services affect only 20 percent of the health status of the population, while the influence of the natural, working, and social environment, and life style, is four times greater. Health status can thus also be *managed* through the environment and life style. Improvement of the environment is a very costly, complex, and lengthy matter. In choosing an optimum utilization of available resources, therefore, it would be valuable to know the relationship between the population health status (with regard to individual nozological units or groups, or as a whole) and the rates and periods of exposure to various risk factors, both individually and combined. This knowledge should be available on both a qualitative and quantitative basis. For the time being, these relationships can be evaluated only with great difficulty or not at all. Integration of systems simulation with the information system outlined above, however, would make this task much easier.

Conclusion

We can give a positive answer to both questions which we posed above. We are justified in using unverified models in support of health care decision-making, in those cases where we can, as yet, verify the adequacy of models only insofar as they correctly interpret hitherto observed data. They represent the best means available. In such case, however, we should draw attention to the fact that the model is unverified and that its use, e.g. for forecasting future developments, can only yield results of a hypothetical nature. We should be aware of the fact that this is, for the time being, the only way, even if a lengthy one, to verify these models. The second approach, which has not yet been fully developed, involves the setting up of national information systems concerning the health status of the population, the state of the environment, etc. Such information systems would open up new possibilities for social medicine and epidemiological research. We need to change the traditional practice of creating such models only for data which are already available, and to develop a new approach along the lines suggested. Only in this way we can ensure that such information systems will, from the beginning, play a proper role in supporting decision-making in the management of health care.

References

1. Kotva M (1987) New version of the agreement on understanding the notion "Simulation of systems". In: Hamata V (ed) Proceedings of the European congress on simulation (September 1987). Academia, Prague, pp 263-266
2. Kotva M (1988) Simulation of biological processes and of health care systems: Methodological Problems. In: Carson ER, Kneppo P, Krekule I (eds) Proceedings of the fourth IMECO Conference. Plenum Press, New York, pp 337-344
3. Dickson D (1988) Perestroika and détente boost IIASA's prospects. Science 241:285-286
4. Lane SM (1988) IIASA's credibility. Science 241 (2):1144
5. Brooks H, McDonald A, Keyfitz N (1988) Support for IIASA. Science 242:495-496

Towards a Comprehensive Health Policy Model

L. Bonneux and J. J. M. Barendregt

Introduction

In most industrialized countries, expenditures in the medical sector have consistently been growing faster than GNP over the past few decades, and the end of this trend is not in sight. On the contrary, exploding medical technology and demographic developments suggest that the trend will accelerate. Consequently, in years to come policy makers in the health sector will increasingly be forced to make choices about the kind and amount of services that will be available. Given this inevitability, it would be beneficial if choices could be made on an informed basis, rather than haphazardly.

Providing relevant information is the primary aim of medical technology assessment. As measures of efficiency, cost-effectiveness ratios and cost-utility ratios are used: these relate the total costs generated by a medical procedure, intervention, or programme, including diagnostic and therapeutic procedures, to the expected benefits: increased life expectancy and/or increased quality of life. They are used as yardsticks, for ranking competing health practices and programmes in order of their relative efficiency.

Methodological Problems

Although medical technology assessment has become an accepted methodology, many problems still have to be considered.

Comparability

The outcomes of different studies cannot easily be compared, because the methodology of these studies has not been standardized.

For the numerator of cost-utility ratios, different definitions of costs are often used. There is still discussion about how productivity losses are to be evaluated, and how and when costs induced by a longer life-span, with its inevitable morbidity, are to be included. As a rule, costs induced by informal care are omitted.

As for the denominator, if the appropriate outcome is to be measured in terms of utilities such as quality adjusted life years (QALY) the problems are even worse. There is a wide array of methods to evaluate health status, most of which are disease-specific, making comparisons between different diseases hazardous. It is far from clear how to evaluate time preferences. Discussions on how to evaluate a very skewed distribution of the quality of life in a population, as a consequence of an intervention, have scarcely begun. For example, a treatment (such as chemotherapy for breast cancer) may cause little or no ill effects in 75% of the population, but be almost tolerable for the remaining 25%. Is a mean, or a median, a fair description of the quality of life of this population?

Effectiveness

Medical effectiveness is difficult to measure. Epidemiologists know how difficult it is to prove any beneficial effect at all, let alone to quantify it within reasonable confidence limits. Without randomized clinical trials (RCT) results depend on observational evidence with data that are poor, often inconsistent, and almost always unclear. RCT are the paradigm of clinical epidemiology, but they are expensive and take a long time, and even with them the follow-up is rarely sufficient to make exact estimates of benefit. Moreover, study populations for RCT are always selected ones, and inference to the *general population of patients*, with a different age distribution, a different mix of severity of illness, and concomitant morbidity cannot be taken for granted.

Multi-Factorial Relationships

The cost-effectiveness of a particular medical intervention for a particular disease should not be measured in isolation from all other diseases and interventions, or from the demographic characteristics of the population. The costs and effects of one intervention depend on assumptions made about the costs and effects of others. For example, the costs and effects of breast cancer screening depend on the efficacy of breast cancer treatment, on the early diagnostic capabilities of mammography, on the general awareness of the public (as a result of health information), etc. The effectiveness of interventions targeted at diseases of old age, such as prostatic cancer, depend largely on assumptions made about life expectancy (and consequently on the mortality rates from other diseases).

Likewise, utilities and costs depend on assumptions made about other morbidity rates. For example, if smoking cessation diverts death from *cheap* causes, such as sudden cardiac death or lung cancer, towards death at a very old age without changing morbidity rates, more *expensive* patients with dementia, invalidity, etc., will result.

Reference Values

In addition to the lack of comparability, these studies lack a baseline of reference values. It is not clear whether the amounts mentioned are too high, average, or a bargain as compared with other medical interventions, whether old or new.

The Concept of a Multi-Disease Environment

A possible approach to a more consistent ranking of competing health practices, and to comparing relative efficiencies, is a large-scale public health model incorporating the most important causes of morbidity and mortality. Standardization is less of a methodological problem, and it is possible to take into account co-existing morbidity, mortality selection, and demographic changes. Such a health policy model is known as TAM (technology assessment methodology).

The aims of TAM are:

- to give a realistic description of public health, health care utilization, and costs, and their developments over time;
- to model the dynamics caused by the evolution of medical technology, demographic changes, changing risk factor distributions in the population, and unexplained secular trends in the epidemiology of the diseases under study;
- to give insight into the relative efficiencies of important existing interventions and sectors of the health care system, which can provide a general framework within which these relative efficiencies can be compared.
- to allow rankings of different interventions and programmes, and to allow priority planning in research and development.

The TAM model is a causal one, built on actual medical knowledge. In a first step, the most important diseases are selected, and their interrelationships are assessed. In a second step, a synthesis of what is known about the epidemiology, natural history, and effective therapy of a specific disease is made. In a third step, a simplified state-transition model, establishing cause-and-effect sequences, is conceived. Finally, these sequences are quantified by using parameters extracted from the large body of international medical literature, and are checked for consistency with the available Dutch data.

The multi-disease model is based on the theory of competing risks. Diseases are modelled in proprietary modules which produce incidence, prevalence, and mortality rates. On the assumption of independence, the crude mortality rates from the disease modules are equal to the net mortality rates, which implies that they are additive [1]. This assumption of independence allows the prevalence rates in the population to be projected, in order to yield the degree of co-morbidity (see Fig.1).

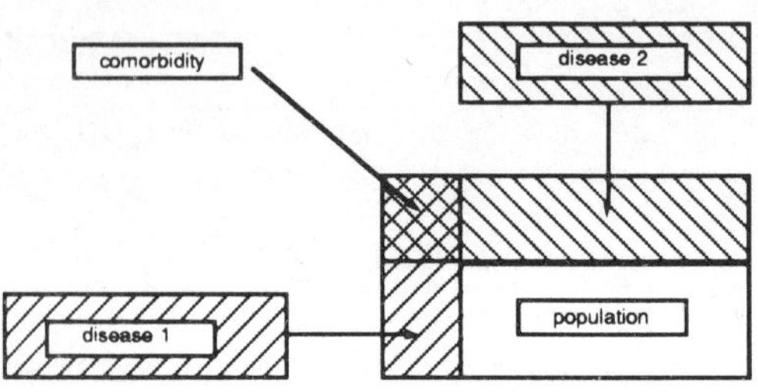

Fig. 1. Comorbidity in a population

We allow for two instances where an assumption of independence is clearly unjustified. One is when two or more diseases have a known common risk factor (for example, smoking is a risk factor for lung cancer and ischaemic heart disease, as well as for several other diseases). The other is when one disease (e.g. diabetes) is a known risk factor for one or more other diseases. In both cases independence, and hence additivity, are conditioned by the prevalence of the risk factor or disease.

TAM incorporates the few risk factors we judge most relevant. The primary aim of incorporating risk factors is not to produce a *second-generation Prevent model* [2], which ranks risk factor interventions by incorporating morbidity, but to allow for heterogeneity in our populations, creating high-risk groups who are at risk for many diseases that cause morbidity and mortality. An example is the cigarette-smoking patient with ischaemic heart disease, on whom we confer a higher risk for cancer and stroke than on his non-smoking counterpart.

Disease history is modelled in as much detail as possible for such a large-scale model. The ultimate aim is to model incidence, recurrences, and prevalence of some thirty diseases and their significant interactions by age, stage, and sex. The choice of diseases is based on their relevance to mortality and/or morbidity. Costs are assigned to incidences and prevalences, and health statuses are evaluated to estimate QALY.

To assign a value to a health status, we need a measure which is not disease-specific. The literature about breast cancer and quality of life [3] includes very few controlled studies, with disparate methodologies. We decided to develop our own measure to evaluate health statuses, based on the concepts of the EUROQOL group [4]. We used published data to estimate the levels of five dimensions of well being: Activities of Daily Life, Mobility, Social Activities, Pain or other Somatic Discomfort, and Anguish or Depression. We related these to the levels in a reference population, and evaluated these ratios in a way which corresponded to the preferences of the reference population.

This measure is necessarily crude, but comparisons with other methods showed that often there were only minor differences, due to the high degree of correlation. Nevertheless, the inherent subjectivity of any quantitative measure of QOL makes sensitivity analyses based on different assumptions necessary.

Face Validity versus Statistical Validity

The single most important problem is the multi-dimensional nature of such a large-scale model. Programming or computing time are lesser constraints than the abundance of assumptions and parameters. We try to restrict our disease states and risk factors as much as possible, but even so the data don't allow a formal estimation. Most parameters are *guesstimates* [5], made by iterative processes of informed guessing based on the available literature, in such a way that results reflect observed incidence, prevalence, survival, and mortality rates where these are available.

Validity cannot be established by formal statistical methods, as there is a wealth of parameters. It is impossible to check each and every assumption that is built into the model; we can only evaluate the aggregate effects. Consequently, there is no independent test of validity of the simplifications and assumptions made [6].

This is a serious dilemma: statistical models [1, 7] can be validated, but depend on so many simplifications that they risk losing medical relevance. State-transition models such as Prevent, TAM, or Weinstein's Coronary Heart Disease Model are easier to understand; they are based on medical evidence and simulate, albeit partially, the complexities of disease processes. Face validity is high, but formal validation is impossible, at least in practice.

Evolution of the Project

Thirty-two disease groups were identified, covering the complete ICD code. Criteria used were high mortality, prevalence, or morbidity rates.

The first group of diseases to be tackled was cancer. The validity of cancer mortality data is well known, cancer registries provide incidence and survival data, and recently a large body of literature on quality of life was published. We use the large database of the Breast Cancer Screening Project group; a breast cancer model is now in operation and publications are being prepared. Breast cancer will serve as a model for all other cancers to be studied.

The second group was cardiovascular diseases, in particular ischaemic heart disease. The latter is an extremely difficult application, as the underlying disease process, atherosclerosis, is virtually impossible to identify, recurring incidences are unpredictable, and therapy depends more on supply (including economic and political constraints) than on objective needs or subjective demands. Numerous assumptions and simplifications need to be made, and even more parameters need to be estimated. Definitions of clinical syndromes, such as angina pectoris (AP) and congestive cardiac heart failure (CHF), are unclear. There are no registries of incident cases, so neither are there population-based survival data. Mortality data, including heterogeneous groups such as sudden death, are less valid than those for cancer. Interactions with risk factors, and other diseases such as diabetes and infectious diseases, are known to exist and probably are important. We use the fundamental concepts of the Coronary Heart Disease Policy Model [8], with somewhat different states (congestive cardiac heart failure is included, and cardiac arrest is omitted) and events (cardiac arrest is replaced by sudden cardiac death, and PTCA, an invasive non-surgical technique to dilate coronary vessels, is included next to coronary artery bypass surgery).

In the meantime, a risk factor model is being conceived to model the interrelationships between different diseases. The necessary marriage between a complex reality and the strict simplifications needed to keep the model manageable still poses severe problems.

Conclusions

It is clear that, in the years to come, policy makers in the health sector will be forced to make choices about the kind and amount of services that will be available. To do so, they will need tools which are reliable and easy to understand. Simulation models may be one answer, but to evaluate old and new health practices and interventions, they need to be based on complex medical knowledge, and this hinders formal testing of the large body of simplifications and assumptions. By structuring common sense and medical evidence in a quantified causal model and by making reasonable assumptions about missing information, such models will not, of course, be able to reproduce the true world, but they may cast light on the many consequences of trends and decisions, thereby assisting health policy makers in making more rational choices.

References

1. Manton KG, Stallard E (1988) Chronic disease modelling. Charles Griffin, London, pp 16-20
2. Gunning-Schepers L (1989) The health benefits of prevention: a simulation approach. Elsevier, Amsterdam, pp 13-66
3. de Haes JCJM, de Koning HJ, van Oortmarssen GJ, van Agt HME, de Bruijn AE, van der Maas PJ (1991) The impact of breast cancer screening programmes on quality-adjusted life-years. Int J Cancer. (in press)
4. Essink-Bot, Bonsel GI, van der Maas PI (1990) Valuation of health states by the general public: feasibility of a standardized measurement procedure. Soc Sci Med 31:1201-1206
5. Wolfson MC (1989) POHEM - A new approach to the estimation of health status adjusted life expectancy. Paper presented to the first workshop of the international network on health expectancy - REVES, September 1989, Quebec. (Unpublished)
6. Weinstein MC (1989) Methodologic issues in policy modelling for cardiovascular disease. J Amer Coll Cardiol 14:38A-43A
7. Woodbury MA, Manton KG (1977) A random walk of human mortality and aging. Theor Popul Biol 11:37-48
8. Weinstein MC, Coxson PG, Williams LW, Pass TM, Stason WB, Goldman L (1987) Forecasting coronary heart disease incidence, mortality and cost: the coronary heart disease policy model. Amer J Publ Hlth 77:1417-1426

Mortality and Morbidity Models - a Review

M. Rusnak

Introduction

This paper reviews methods and models developed for health status analysis. It aims to identify and demonstrate results from scholars of different origins and backgrounds. It is intended not as an exhaustive summary of published material, but as an indication of current trends. Selected topics are discussed with regard to the application of models which have been developed. The methodology itself, as well as a precise mathematical description, is beyond the scope of this paper. Nevertheless, some basic classification has been applied with the aim of showing different methods of building a model. The paper deals with problems related to chronic noncommunicable diseases and their effects on the health care system. Communicable diseases and acute conditions have been described in other scientific contributions, and thus are not included in this paper. However, the author is aware of their developments and achievements in this field, and of the influence of current work on the author's field of interest.

A Systems Approach to Health Care

The health care system is considered as a large and complex dynamic system. It consists of a set of interrelated subsystems, closely tied to external systems and joined by a common goal: the health of the population. Such a system also comprises several hierarchical levels. Venedictov and Chigan [1] identified some specific and nonspecific problems of a systems approach to health care. The former are concerned with the content of information for the components of each level. The latter cover all levels of the system, and relationships with external systems. A functional description of the health care system was given by Kiselev [2]. While it seems too complicated to be used in solving real health problems, it could be useful for the education of students and young health care professionals.

A more pragmatic approach has been adopted by Gibbs [3] with his model, which is designed for planning health care resources. Several models are based on his particular scheme. Some other approaches have been used in analyzing health care systems. Van der Werff [4] describes different health care system structures. In addition, he outlines possible strategies for health care system management, as well as differences between various countries. He provides an in-depth analysis of systems, based on an extensive knowledge of the data. Understanding health care as a system facilitates the introduction of formal methods of analysis.

Disease Prevalence Models

Although this paper is not concerned with communicable diseases, models of acute bacterial diseases should be mentioned in order to stress the notion of continuity of human knowledge. In 1978, WHO [5] published an overview of existing epidemiological models of communicable diseases. Since then, models of AIDS have taken up most attention. However, the methodology used in the models described is still topical. The WHO booklet is also worth reading by anyone with an interest in the modelling of noncommunicable diseases.

Knowledge of indices, such as the incidence and prevalence of chronic degenerative diseases, is a basic tool for managers of health care. Planning and controlling of health care depend on the availability of appropriate data. In many countries, however, such data are often lacking. The only way to develop models for estimating levels and trends of incidence and prevalence rates in a population is to use such data as are available, or to rely on an expert estimate (or both). Different approaches are possible for different purposes.

Coronary heart disease is a multi-stage disease of substantial interest to clinicians, epidemiologists, and other health specialists. The risk factors are to some extent known, and various new surveys are being carried out. Different teams are trying to quantify the risk from cigarette smoking, hypertension, serum cholesterol, etc. A patient's progression from one disease stage to another is measured by the severity of the disease, such as the amount of myocardial damage. Based on these observable quantities Wolf et al. [6] derived a model of coronary disease prevalence. It consists of three disease stages: angina, infarct, and re-infarct. The sum of the prevalence of each stage is the total prevalence for coronary disease. The population at risk is divided between these stages, and flow is assumed between the stages. The introduction of antihypertensive medication is simulated by a step decrease in the rates of inflow to the next disease stage among the population in risk. The magnitude of the steps varied between 10% and 50%. Rate parameters and subgroup sizes were taken from the literature, and the system was assumed to be in equilibrium prior to intervention. The authors hypothesized that the introduction of effective antihypertensive medication in the late sixties was the sole disturbance introduced into the system. Although this assumption obviously ignores other major changes that occurred in primary prevention and treatment, it is justified for the purpose of this investigation. The results indicate that the time constants of coronary heart disease are large enough to produce a noticeable change in mortality over a period of about ten years, if the disturbance is introduced in a stepwise fashion. Results suggest that the presently observed decline in mortality may conceivably be due to an isolated phenomenon, such as the adoption of a new procedure. The authors further suggest that, because of the long time constants of the system and the continuous introduction of new preventive measures, the system will rarely be in equilibrium, and thus the effects of planned interventions must be distinguished from changes occurring in the system due to disturbances preceding the study period. The authors do not provide a more detailed description of model formulation or available data. Nevertheless, their approach seems a promising one.

Based on the general model for degenerative diseases developed by Klementiev [7] scientists from the Istituto Superiore di Sanita in Rome, Italy, designed an approach to the estimation of chronic diseases morbidity. They estimated cardiovascular diseases morbidity using mortality data from the Italian areas of the Seven Countries Study [8]. The model used comprises four sections: healthy people, sick people, and deaths from non-cardiovascular and cardiovascular causes. Using mortality rates and survival data as inputs for the model, the incidence rates were estimated. The number of deaths, population data, and survival data were used as model inputs. The prevalence and incidence of myocardial infarction in Italian males over a decade (1969-79) was calculated. The generally good agreement between estimated and observed rates indicates that the model's hypotheses about population structure and the chronic nature of the disease may be applied in practice.

A similar approach was adopted by the same group for estimating cancer morbidity [9]. They estimated the incidence and prevalence of cancers in the Varese province using the official data for people resident in that province in 1976 and 1977. Survival data for cancers were not available in Italy, and the authors referred to published American data [10]. The results obtained proved the correctness of the model in this particular application.

A different approach to estimating the prevalence of cardiovascular disease was used by a group of scholars from Adaptive Resource Policies, at IIASA. In March 1982, the Slovakian Deputy Minister of Health requested the IIASA team to work with a group of Slovak medical specialists on a preliminary assessment of health problems related to the environment. A workshop took place in April 1983 at the Research Institute of Medical Bionics, Bratislava, which has subsequently collaborated with the IIASA on an extension of the work. Out of that meeting came a model that quantifies theories about the relationships between environmental factors and the incidence of hypertension and diabetes.

The model [11] is split into two submodels, dealing with risk group population and heart disease population. The first includes three risk groups (health, hypertensive, and diabetic), from which the annual incidence of heart disease is calculated. Using annual incidence data, the heart disease prevalence and other indices are calculated. These data were used for subsequent estimations. Diabetes prevalence and incidence were estimated by expert opinion. The same approach was adopted for the estimation of several transition factors as well. The model was designated to allow the participants to examine several health care management scenarios, and to study their consequences. The results confirmed the feasibility of developing simulation models to facilitate joint analysis of public health problems by teams of policy makers, physicians, and other specialists drawn from different levels of the health care hierarchy. The meeting also demonstrated that the quick development of computer models can break down communication barriers and focus attention on alternatives to existing health care policies.

The IIASA Population Group, in cooperation with medical doctors, has developed several other models of chronic diseases prevalence. These models are more sophisticated than the one just mentioned, and are based on data from health surveys. The model of Chronic Pulmonary Disease (COPD) prevalence estimation [12] consists of two major blocks of logic: population development and COPD risk factors development. The population is divided into the following three groups: healthy individuals, those at risk of COPD, and those suffering from COPD. The risk group covers three types of risk for COPD: cigarette smoking, air pollution, and frequent respiratory infections. The model provides forecasts of COPD morbidity, and permits the testing of different scenarios on the effects of preventive measures applied.

The model on lung cancer morbidity forecasts was developed later [13]. Its structure is similar to the previous one, but the number of risk groups was reduced to one: smokers. The model distinguishes among non-smokers, current smokers, and quitters. All data are stratified according to sex and age-groups. The main aim of this model is to predict future developments in lung cancer morbidity. For this purpose, forecasts of risk factors were made as well. The model was run under several scenarios. The authors tried to highlight the impact of preventive measures in terms of reducing the population at risk by changing transition coefficients. The model offers a user-friendly environment: it stores data in database format, and produces results in graphic and tabular form.

The Dynamic Morbidity Model (DYMOD) is another member of the family of morbidity models. In estimating morbidity rates for a population with a changing age structure, it is necessary to describe the *destiny* of sick individuals from the beginning of illness to death, as in demographic models. That is why the cohort approach, along with the state-space approach, was chosen to describe disease dynamics. The precise mathematical description, as well as program and files specification, can be found in Kitsul [14]. The model was tested on data for cancer at several sites and from different countries. For comparison of cancer trends in Poland and Czechoslovakia, the model was used by Rusnak and Bojanczyk [15].

Different models were designed based on statistical modelling approaches. The one described by Testa et al. [16] was developed to evaluate trends in age and period of diagnosis, and to identify differences in these trends with regard to qualitative variables such as sex and tumor site. Parameter estimates were obtained through a weighted least squares procedure, and hypothesis testing was carried out using minimum modified chi-squared statistics. These procedures were applied to colon cancer incidence rates for Connecticut males and females during the period 1940-74. Using mathematical models of cancer incidence rates for substantive analysis can be useful for generating hypotheses in cancer epidemiology. Such modelling proves worthwhile because it allows the investigator to summarize the trends and patterns of cancer incidence through model parameters, which then may be tested statistically for the purpose of identifying significant effects of independent variables.

Logistic regression models have been used by various authors for describing disease processes. The one by Brown and Chu [17] is based on the Armitage-Doll [18] model of the carcinogenic process, for use in analyzing epidemiologic case-control studies of cancer. These methods aim to provide inferences regarding the stage or stages in the cancer process at which a particular influence acts. The example provided by the authors shows evidence that carcinogens in cigarette smoke affect the transition rates for two separate stages in the development of lung cancer, and the relative magnitudes of these effects are estimated. The data for this analysis came from a European multi-center case-control study of lung cancer.

Another example of the use of a statistical model is described by Stevens and Moolgavkar [19]. The authors estimated attributable and relative risks of lung cancer according to cigarette smoking status. Data on cigarette consumption were related to mortality rates in order to estimate time trends in rates, and the relation of age to risk in non-smokers. Trends in non-smokers reflect environmental influences that have been masked in the overall rates by the strong effect of tobacco.

Several works of this type have been published by Manton et al. A review of methods used was submitted to WHO for publication in 1986 [20]. The recently published book [21] covers the main types of chronic diseases models. Major emphasis is put on selecting the most appropriate model for a given data set, and tailoring that model to fit the special features of those data. Detailed numerical examples are presented for all models. The final chapter discusses issues in extrapolating the results of a given analysis to the general population and to future years. The methodologies of single- and multi-state life-table models, event models with time censoring, mixed continuous and discrete-state models, stochastic compartment models, and nonparametric multivariate pattern-recognition models are discussed in detail. The book is ideal for an introduction to the quantitative epidemiology of chronic noncommunicable diseases.

A model for estimating diabetes prevalence, designed by Hauser [22], includes nine stages of disease. The results were used for estimating diabetes prevalence in Bohemia.

Several other approaches are used to analyze, estimate, and project morbidity of noncommunicable diseases. The ones described above are intended to emphasize two points:

- the role of the specialist (clinician, epidemiologist) in model design, verification, and applications;
- data availability and methods of data collection, and their effect on the success of any model.

The application of a model is affected less by its mathematical description than by the available data. Several models created by mathematicians have never reached the stage of being applied to real data. Simple models with a clear structure are frequently more useful than complex and sophisticated ones. The user interface also plays an important role.

Resource Allocation Models

Models of morbidity represent a substantial proportion of health care resources models. The estimation of resources needs is based on a morbidity forecast, as for example in the case of hospital beds estimation [3]:

$$\frac{\text{hospital beds} \cdot \text{morbidity} \cdot \text{hospitalization rate} \cdot \text{average length of stay}}{\text{occupancy}}$$

where *occupancy* equals the average number of days per year a bed can be occupied. This calculation can be performed for each type of disease, and by summation the need for each resource can be estimated.

As the reader may have noticed, in evaluating morbidity due to noncommunicable diseases, problems usually arise in connection with data availability, whereas in resources models data are available from routine statistics. The methods of data processing, and approaches used, stem from widely used mathematical and statistical approaches (simplex problem, linear programming, regression analysis). All kinds of methods have been used for different purposes in various countries. However, only a few countries employ people to use these methods in planning. A review of health care models published up to the year 1977 has been compiled by Fleissner and Klementiev [23]. An exhaustive overview of planning health delivery systems can be found in other publications [24].

Klementiev and Chigan designed model AMER as an aggregated model for evaluating resource requirements in a health care system. It integrates estimations of the following types of resources: total number of beds, total number of inpatient doctor equivalents, and total number of outpatient doctor equivalents. The model structure consists, in this context, of four main blocks: population, morbidity, standards, and resource requirements. A hypothesis was put forward about the future evolution of fertility and death rates. The population forecast is based on these rates, and general morbidity is calculated. Calculations of hospital bed requirements are based on average length of stay, percent hospitalization, and bed occupancy. The result, multiplied by the number of beds per inpatient doctor equivalent, yields inpatient doctor equivalent requirements. The outpatient doctor equivalent requirements are determined using data about morbidity, workload, and number of consultations per episode. The model is designed to help decision-makers to test different policy options, and to select the best among them. Forecasting of mortality and morbidity trends is supported by the model as well. A hidden source of difficulties is often the estimation of total morbidity, a fact which may explain why few attempts have been made to apply AMER in the planning process.

The wider application of desegregated models is determined by data availability. The Desegregated Resource Allocation Model (DRAM) is a behavioural model designed to simulate how the health care system allocates limited supplies of resources between competing demands. The output of the model represents the number of people cared for in each treatment group, and within each group the distribution between alternative forms of care. The model also gives the level of resources allocated to each person. The model and its theoretical basis have been formulated and discussed by Gibbs [25]. The model assumes, firstly, that there are never enough resources to satisfy all demands made on the health care service; and secondly, that the aggregate behaviour of the health care service can be represented by a unity function whose parameters can be inferred from past resource allocations. The model has been successfully tested on data from different countries, among them the UK [26] and Czechoslovakia [27].

Another model, called RAMOS, considers the interactions between resource supply and demand, but at a geographical level. More specifically, this model has been designed to explore the effects on hospitalization rates and patient flow patterns, in a region or a country, resulting from changes over time in the number and location of hospital beds, the population size and structure, the relative morbidity, the rate at which hospitals are able to treat patients, and the availability and efficiency of transport services and car travel [28]. The model used is a behavioural one, and is of the singly-constrained gravity kind. It argues that patient flows from an area are in proportion to the difficulty of geographical access in terms of travel time or distance. The model operates in two distinct modes: a calibration mode and a forecasting mode. The results obtained showed that the gravity model approach has considerable potential, both in decision-making and in forecasting the resulting demands on health care services when resource supply and population structure are changing simultaneously over space. Similar models are now in use in other European countries [29, 30].

The goal of the TAMS model [31] is to estimate the number and allocation of specialized medical services over a given territory. The model employs modified M-median of weighted graph method for optimal allocation of the services. The authors ran the model for twelve centres with ECG screening capabilities. The results suggested that ECG allocation between district catchment areas was sufficiently accurate. This has been agreed on by health care managers from the region.

Manpower Models

Another frequent application of models is manpower planning. It can be summarized as follows. First, the planner must assess the demand for manpower that a service organized in a particular way would generate. Then, the supply that could meet the demand is in general an iterative process, which stops when an acceptable plan is reached. In such a plan, supply will match demand, at least within tolerable limits. The demand itself would be the manpower part of a complete set of resources designed to give an acceptable service.

A multi-state manpower projection model is described by Pelling [32]. It allows a planner to make year-by-year projections of numbers by grade, by time in grade, and by age, sex, and region of origin. It is possible to fix the growth rate for any grade, and thereby to represent a demand profile. Thus the effect on the manpower system of setting a demand target, with a given supply trend, can be investigated. For medical manpower, separate specialties can be examined. In other manpower systems, analogous divisions may occur. If the model is used for this purpose, stocks and inter-specialty flows must be defined with care. In the lower grades, for instance, it may be difficult to assign a doctor to a particular specialty. The model has been successfully tested on data from the UK.

Ghosh [33] has published a model for health manpower forecasting for India. The publication comprises an overview of approaches used by different authors. Similar models were published by various other authors [34, 35]. Standridge et al. [36, 37] constructed a simulation model of medical manpower for the State of Indiana. It took into account four elements: primary care physicians, the volume of services provided, the population, and the volume of services demanded. The model projected these variables for future years, based on an understanding of the process affecting the values of the variables.

Dental manpower requirements were the subject of a systems dynamics study by Hirsch and Killingsworth [38]. Of special interest in this simulation was the focus on improving oral health, rather than on increasing the number of dental visits.

The supply, demand, and distribution of nurses was the subject of Bergan and Hirsch's systems dynamics model [39]. Four sectors were modelled: education, employment, demand, and demography, with seven possible employment settings and five levels of educational preparation, to estimate the impact of changes in programs and policies on nursing personnel. The model was used to predict nursing personnel behaviour under various conditions, over a four-year time frame.

Conclusion

We have reviewed above the following items:

- models for morbidity estimations and projections;
- models for health care resource allocation;
- models for manpower planning.

Naturally these activities are interrelated and interdependent, but clearly each is required to perform a specialized task. Most methods described are of interest from the application point of view. In order to start applying them, the following points must be taken into consideration:

- potential users and their willingness to use them;
- model availability;
- available data, feasibility to use data from other sources, and form of data;
- conditions under which each model might be distributed.

The crucial point in applying models to real-life situations is to find potential users. When a person is not convinced of the fact that he needs a particular model to help him in his work, he will never use it. He must become acquainted with the power of the model. Bearing in mind the applications, the following points must be considered:

- who are the potential users, and how willing are they to use these methods?
- what models are at a stage that allows for their immediate use?
- what data are available, and what transformations must be made before introducing them into models?
- what are the conditions for distributing models in Europe?

A promising approach to convince potential users was a workshop organized by IIASA for health care managers in Czechoslovakia. Several events of this kind, organized in various countries, could attract the attention of health care managers. Before organizing such a workshop, a preliminary model or models, as well as data for a particular country, should be prepared. The use of a microcomputer for this purpose is desirable. The demonstration and model construction may be based on some existing models or software.

Preparation of an inventory of models, model designers, and model users is important and a questionnaire sent to people who are known to be working in this area can help to achieve this. The questionnaire could be adapted from the one published by Fleissner and Klementiev [23] in order to include older models and prepare a document for WHO. Queries on available data should also be included. Through such an approach, it might be possible to map the situation of health care system modelling in Europe.

In order to encourage health system policy makers to use models, one should start with a very simple approach. One way would be to prepare a book of simple exploratory projections for all European countries. The projected data should characterize the health care system in each country, and the trend of its future development. Another important task is to continue work on models of morbidity, resource allocation, and manpower. In order to identify possible new approaches, the following facts should be borne in mind:

- Current models deal with only a small number of risk factors which usually include smoking or hypertension. The real situation is more complicated, however, and models which deal with multiple risk factors are much closer to reality. From the viewpoint of data collection, such models require much effort to include a wide range of risk factors, because information on the interaction of risk factors is still incomplete. There is also a shortage of data on environmental risk factors. Existing models would need to be redesigned, and demand for computer memory would increase.

- Existing models are designed for the user who has a good background in mathematics, statistics, and computing. They need to be redesigned for the health policy maker, with emphasis given to the user interface. This applies to all the above-mentioned models.
- With health care managers in mind as the primary users of models, possibilities of educating them in their use need to be created. Existing WHO courses (in London and Moscow) could be used for this purpose. Using existing models as examples, participants could be taught the basic principles of model construction, data pre-processing, how to run models, and how to interpret results. Teachers should be found who can explain the principles without introducing too much formal mathematics, and who have experience of teaching medical doctors.

References

1. Venediktov DD, Chigan EN (1977) The IIASA health care systems model. In: Chigan EN (ed) Systems modelling in health care. IIASA, Laxenburg, p 112
2. Kiselev AS (1975) Methodological problems of constructing a health care macro-model. In: Venediktov DD (ed) Health system modelling and the information system for the coordination of research in oncology (Proceedings of the IIASA biomedical conference). IIASA, Laxenburg, p 564
3. Gibbs RJ (1977) The components of the IIASA health care system model. In: Chigan EN (ed) Systems modelling in health care. IIASA, Laxenburg, p 112
4. van der Werff A (1976) Organizing health care systems, a developmental approach. Greve Offset B.V., Endhoven, p 279
5. Cvjetanovic B, Grab K, Uemura K (1978) Dynamics of acute bacterial diseases. World Health Organization, Geneva, p 143
6. Wolf HK, Gregor RD, MacKenzie, RB Rautaharju P (1984) An epidemiological model for coronary heart disease (CHD). In: van Eimeren W, Engelbrecht R, Flagle CD (eds) Proceedings of the third international conference on system science in health care. Springer, Berlin Heidelberg New York, p 485
7. Klementiev A (1977) On the estimation of morbidity. IIASA, Laxenburg, RM-77-043, pp 1-23
8. Verdecchia A, Capocaccia R, Mariotti S (1984) Estimation of cardiovascular diseases morbidity using mortality data. In: von Eimeren W, Engelbrecht R, Flagle CD (eds) Proceedings of the third international conference on system science in health care. Springer, Berlin Heidelberg New York, p 485

9. Verdecchia A, Capocaccia R, Mazzoni C (1985) Estimation of cancer morbidity using mortality data. Tumori 71:431-439
10. US Department of Health and Human Services (1976) Cancer patient survival. Report no. 5 NHI publication 81, p 992
11. Koonce JF, Yashin AI, Walters CJ, Rusnak M (1984) Modelling of public health: Call for interdisciplinary actions. IIASA, Laxenburg, p 47
12. Rusnak M, Yashin A, Kristufek P (1985) The future of lung diseases: COPD model for Slovakia. IIASA, Laxenburg, CP-85-49
13. Rusnak M, Yashin A, Merinska I (1986) Smoking and lung cancer prevalence: Slovakian case study. IIASA, Laxenburg, CP-86-12, p 40
14. Kitsul PI (1980) A dynamic approach to the estimation of morbidity. IIASA, Laxenburg, WP-80-71, pp 1-30
15. Rusnak M, Bojanczyk M (1983) On the estimation of prevalence for neoplastic disease in Czechoslovakia and Poland. Medical Bionics Research Institute, Bratislava, pp 1-12
16. Testa MA, Meigs L, Flannery JT (1980) Mathematical modelling of cancer incidence rates: linear models of colon cancer in Connecticut. J Chron Dis 33:733-743
17. Brown CC, Chu KC (1987) Use of multi-stage models to infer stage affected by carcinogenic exposure: example of lung cancer and cigarette smoking. J Chron Dis 40 (Suppl 2):171S-179S
18. Armitage P, Doll R (1954) The age distribution of cancer and a multi-stage theory of carcinogenesis. Brit J Cancer 8:1-12
19. Stevens RG, Moolgavkar SH (1984) A cohort analysis of lung cancer and smoking in British males. Amer J Epidemiol 119 (4):624-641
20. Manton KG (1986) Compartment model approaches for estimating the paramet process under changing risk factors exposure. Comput Biom Res 19:151-169
21. Manton KG, Stallard E (1988) Chronic diseases modelling: measurement and evaluation of the risks of chronic diseases process. Charles Griffin, London and Oxford University Press, New York, p 279
22. Rusnak M, Hauser F, Kotva M (1988) Models of chronic non-infectious diseases. Cs. zdravotnictvi 36 (1):15-28
23. Fleissner P, Klementiev A (1977) Health care system models: a review. IIASA, Laxenburg, RM-77-049, p 99
24. Roberts SD, England WL (1981) Survey of the application of simulation to health care. Simulation series 10 (1):7-19
25. Gibbs RJ (1978) The IIASA health care resource allocation submodel, Mark I. IIASA, Laxenburg, RR-78-008, pp 1-43
26. Aspden P (1980) The IIASA health care resource allocation submodel: DRAM calibration for data from the South-West Health Region. IIASA, Laxenburg, p 22
27. Aspden P, Mayhew L, Rusniak M (1981) DRAM, a model of health care resource allocation in Czechoslovakia. Omega 9 (5):509-518

28. Mayhew L, Taket AR (1980) RAMOS: a model of health care resource allocation in space. IIASA, Laxenburg, WP-80-125, p 56
29. Taket AR (1989) Equity and access: exploring the effects of hospital location on the population served. Journal of the Operational Research Society 40 (11):1001-1009
30. Stone J (1984) Predicting patient flows to local acute hospitals. In: van Eimeren W, Engelbrecht R, Flagle CD (eds) Proceedings of the third international conference on system science in health care. Springer, Berlin Heidelberg New York, pp 1013-1016
31. Rusnak M, Melotova J, Smolak L (1983) Territorial allocation of medical services: Model TAMS. In: Proceedings of the fourth world conference on medical informatics. North Holland, Amsterdam, pp 255-257
32. Pelling M (1982) A multi-state manpower projection model. IIASA, Laxenburg, p 37
33. Ghosh B (1981) Study of health manpower in selected specialities and super-specialities: a long-term perspective for Karnataka. Indian Institute of Management, Bangalore, p 76
34. Meyer M, Grutz M (1982). Health Economics Research Group, Erlangen-Nürnberg, p 63
35. Doyle TC (1974) An analysis of health manpower models. Vol I and II. Vector Research Inc., Ann Arbor, p 112
36. Standridge CR, Pritsker AA, Delcher HD (1978) Issues in the development of a model for planning health manpower. Simulation (July 1978):9-12
37. Standridge CR (1979) Using simulation in health manpower planning. Simuletter 10 (4): 60-62
38. Hirsch GB, Killingsworth WR (1975) A new framework for projecting dental manpower requirements. Inquiry 12 (2):126-142
39. Bergan TA, Hirsch GB (1976) Analysis and planning for improved distribution of nursing personnel and services: a national model of supply, demand, and distribution. Pugh-Roberts Associates Inc., Cambridge Mass., p 125

Estimation of Morbidity from Chronic Disease Mortality

R. Capocaccia

Introduction

Analyzing the impact of chronic degenerative disease on a population often requires simultaneous consideration of mortality and morbidity statistics. However, incidence, prevalence, and mortality are seldom analyzed jointly in the epidemiological literature. This is probably due to the varied availability and reliability of specific information, as well as to the different data sources and collection methods.

The availability of population-based survival data allows for the use of official mortality statistics for the estimation of morbidity levels. Based on the fact that incidence, survival, and mortality are three different aspects of the same morbid process, several methods have been proposed [1-5] to estimate patterns of unobserved morbidity from observed mortality data.

This approach has two advantages. First, from a descriptive point of view, it allows for an analysis of disease trends apart from the effect of changes in patient survival which, in fact, affect mortality rates. Second, in a health care setting, it provides incidence and prevalence estimates of direct utility in the calculation of resource needs.

The potential applications of the method, as well as the most relevant problems it raises, have been extensively discussed elsewhere [5]. The present work aims to show how incidence models can be implemented once survival and official mortality data are known. The equations relating to mortality and morbidity rates are presented both in their more general form and in a reduced form, derived under a few simplifying assumptions. Two different methods for estimating morbidity figures, direct calculations and maximum likelihood estimation, are discussed, along with a review of various incidence models potentially suitable for statistical estimation. Finally, an application of both estimation methods to cancer mortality data in the Italian population is presented.

The Mortality - Morbidity Equations

The relationships between mortality and morbidity in chronic degenerative diseases can be formalized by two mathematical expressions. For this purpose, consider individuals who belong to a same birth cohort. The incidence hazard and prevalence ratio at age x are indicated as $I(x)$ and $N(x)$, respectively; $B(t,x)$ and $D(t,x)$ are the general- and specific-cause death hazard, respectively, at age x for sick individuals diagnosed at age t. Finally, $G(x)$ and $M(x)$ are given to be the general- and specific-cause death hazards in the entire cohort at age x. It can be shown [6] that, for non-reversible diseases, the following system of two integral equations relates incidence and prevalence experienced by the cohort to its own mortality and survival rates:

$$M(x) = \int_0^x (1-N(t))\, I(t)\, D(t,x)\, e^{-\int_t^x (B(t,u)-G(u))\,du}\, dt$$

$$N(x) = \int_0^x (1-N(t))\, I(t)\, e^{-\int_t^x (B(t,u)-G(u))\,du}\, dt\,. \tag{1}$$

These expressions are the basic equations of the mortality/morbidity model presented in this paper. The model does not need assumptions about migrations or population structure, such as stability or lack of mobility. The most relevant assumption required so far is about disease irreversibility; a new case is assumed to remain in the sick status until he or she dies. The model is therefore suitable for many practical applications and for a wide spectrum of pathologies. Such a generality is, however, not always necessary. Sometimes the disease process can also be satisfactorily captured by simpler models, owing either to its own features or to our incomplete knowledge of the process. In these cases, the above equations can be reduced into a simpler form under some further assumptions. In particular, suppose that: (a) the risks of death for the specific cause and for the other causes are independent; (b) the prevalence is low; and (c) the difference $B(t,x) - G(x)$, which represents the increased hazard of sick individuals with respect to the general population, is a function of disease duration x - t alone:

$$B(t,x) - G(x) = C(x - t)\,.$$

If, starting from the differential hazard $C(x\text{-}t)$, we define a death density function:

$$F(x - t) = C(x - t)\, e^{-\int_0^{x-t} C(u)\,du}$$

then it can be shown [6] that the system (1) becomes:

$$M(x) = \int_0^x I(t)\, F(x - t)\, dt$$

$$N(x) = \int_0^x I(t)\, \left(1 - \int_0^{x-t} F(u)\, du\right) dt \;. \tag{2}$$

The first equation is a particular case of the Volterra equation of the first kind, and it has a unique solution for $I(x)$. This equation can now be separately solved by analytic or numerical methods. Once $I(x)$ is obtained, it becomes straightforward to compute $N(x)$ from the second equation. The model does not need assumptions about population stability or lack of mobility. In the following paragraph, a particular analytic solution of equations (2) will be presented.

Morbidity Estimation Methods

The equation system (1) allows one, in principle, to compute incidence and prevalence of each birth cohort once its mortality and survival rates are known. The main difficulty of this approach lies in the availability of the data requested. Looking at the equations (1), it can be seen that cohort mortality data at all previous ages are needed in order to compute incidence and prevalence at a given age x. Most chronic disease cases occur at ages over 60 years, and very seldom is such a lengthy time series of mortality data effectively available.

The situation is illustrated on the Lexis diagram shown in Figure 1. Here, time is represented on the horizontal axis, and age on the vertical axis. Birth cohorts move, while aging, on diagonal lines from the lower-left to the upper-right. Usually, mortality data are available for all ages within a given calendar time interval. In the Figure 1, this interval is represented by the segment AB,

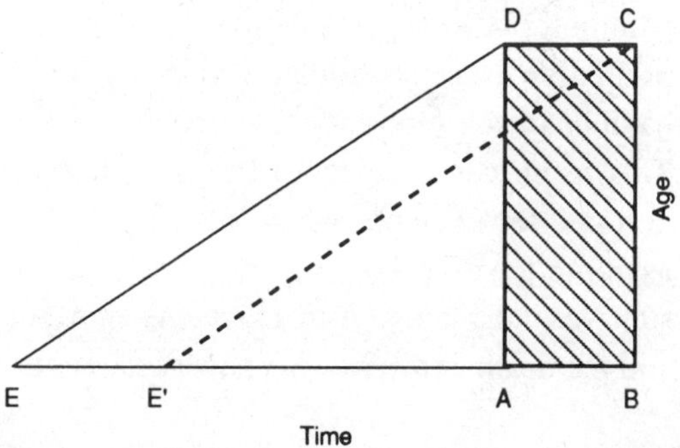

Fig. 1. Lexis diagram of age-time regions in which mortality data would be necessary for a general solution of the morbidity-mortality equation system (white area) and in which they are usually available (shadowed area)

and the rectangle ABCD indicates the region of data availability. Incidence and prevalence at time A (or at time B) of the cohorts crossing the line AD (or BC) can be directly computed from equations (1) only when starting from mortality data in the whole area EAD (or E'BC).

Direct Solution Approach

The problem of data availability can be overcome by starting from the simpler model (2), if relative survival for the specific disease can be assumed as exponential. In this case, we have indeed:

$$F(t) = \lambda\, e^{-\lambda t}$$

and, under the initial conditions $M(0) = M'(0) = 0$, the first equation can be solved in terms of $I(x)$ deriving both sides. The function $N(x)$ is then easily obtained from the second equation by substitution, and we have the solution:

$$I(x) = M(x) + \frac{1}{\lambda}\frac{d}{dx} M(x)$$

$$N(x) = \frac{M(x)}{\lambda} .$$

The expressions state that, if survival is exponential, and under the assumptions leading to the equation system (2), incidence at each age x is given by the mortality level at x plus the derivative of mortality at x divided by the survival parameter λ. The prevalence is given by the mortality divided by λ. In this particular case, morbidity levels can be directly derived from the local behaviour of the mortality function, and retrospective data are no longer needed. This result can be extended to include more general classes of survival distributions, for example when the relative survival curve tends toward a positive asymptotic value 1-A (this happens when a fraction 1-A of the sick individuals survives long enough to reach the mortality level of the general population), and the death density of the new cases is given by a defective exponential:

$$F(t) = A\ \lambda\, e^{-\lambda t} . \tag{3}$$

It is easy to show that, in this case, the following expression for the incidence function is obtained:

$$I(x) = \frac{1}{A}\ M(x) + \frac{1}{\lambda A}\ \frac{d}{dx}\ M(x) . \tag{4}$$

The corresponding expression for prevalence is more complicated, and is a function of the past mortality rates experienced by the cohort:

$$N(x) = \frac{M(x)}{\lambda A} + \frac{1 - A}{\lambda A} \int_0^x M(t)\, dt \ .$$

Maximum Likelihood Approach

A different approach for deriving morbidity values from mortality data is based on statistical estimation [3, 5]. The incidence is assumed to be a regular function of age and other covariates. A maximum likelihood estimation of its parameters is then carried out using equation system (1) to fit observed mortality data.

Let $I(x, t, z, \Theta)$ indicate incidence as a function of age x, time t, a vector of covariates z, and of a set of parameters Θ. If we assume that survival rates are known, we can compute theoretical mortality by means of equation system (1), as a function $M(x, t, \Theta)$ of the parameters Θ in the region ABCD represented in Figure 1.

In practice, mortality and population data are arranged in discrete age classes and time periods. Suppose, then, that the region ABCD is divided into a grid defined by I single-year age classes and P calendar years. If the probability of observing Y_{ip} deaths from n_{ip} person-years at risk can be assumed to be Poisson distributed with expectation $n_{ip} M(x_i, t_p, \Theta)$ and $x_i = i - 0.5$ $t_p = p - 0.5$, then the maximum likelihood estimates of Θ can be obtained by an iteratively weighted least squares procedure [7], maximizing with respect to Θ the expression:

$$w_{ip} \ (Y_{ip} - n_{ip} M(x_i, t_p, \Theta))^2 \tag{5}$$

where the weights w_{ip} are the inverse of the variance of Y_{ip}:

$$w_{ip} = (n_{ip} M(x_i, t_p, \Theta))^{-1}$$

and are recomputed at each step of the procedure.

Methods for statistical estimation of mathematical models of mortality data are of course well known, and appear widely in the epidemiological and demographic literature. Many of these studies rely upon Poisson assumptions, and are based on minimization of expressions such as expression (5). The equation system (2), and the availability of survival data, permit a backward step on the causal chain leading to death, connecting mortality data with incidence models.

In this way, indicators of risk exposure could be related to the onset of illness (the primary event) rather than to death (the final event). Moreover, it would be possible to analyze disease trends and patterns stripped of any interference from factors affecting survival.

Modelling the Incidence Function

The definition of a mathematical function modelling disease incidence is, of course, of primary importance in the estimation procedure. In order to avoid excessive computing time, the number of model parameters must be kept as low as possible. This discourages the use of categorical or dummy variables. Continuous functions of age, time, and other covariates are then considered.

Age is generally the most important variable to be included in the model. For some chronic diseases, as for many tumours, the shape of the relationship between age and incidence derives from theoretical arguments. In the multi-stage theory of carcinogenesis, a tumour is assumed to develop when m mutations have occurred in a single cell. In this case, the age trend of incidence can be expressed by the relation:

$$I(x) = \Theta_1 (x - d)^{m-1} \qquad (6)$$

where d indicates the mean time between tumour onset and diagnosis. The expression (6) appears as a linear relation when it is represented on a double logarithmic scale.

A different type of model, which is not based on biological consideration but which has the advantage of a greater generality, is given by polynomials on the logarithmic or logistic scale:

$$log\,(I(x)) \text{ or } logit\,(I(x)) = \Theta_0 + \Theta_1 x + \Theta_2 x^2 + \cdots\,. \qquad (7)$$

The power of the highest order term must, in this case, be determined by statistical testing of a series of increasing order nested models.

The time trend of the disease can be analyzed by means of two different variables: year of diagnosis (period) and year of birth (cohort). Very few diseases are known in which a reasonable model of incidence dynamics can be stated *a priori* in terms of period or cohort. Expressions like (7) are therefore the most appropriate to model the relationships between these variables and incidence hazard. Assuming that the relative risks (or the odds ratios) attributed to age x, period y, and cohort z combine with each other in a multiplicative way, we can formulate a general age, period, and cohort model:

$$\textit{log } I \text{ or } \textit{logit } I = \Theta_0 + \sum_i \Theta_{1i}\, x^i + \sum_j \Theta_{2j}\, y^j + \sum_k \Theta_{3k}\, z^k \tag{8}$$

where the order of the polynomials must be determined by means of a standard stepwise procedure.

Models like (8) can also be extended to include other known risk indicators. For example, the relationships between parity and female breast cancer incidence can be explored replacing the variable *cohort* in the model with a factor expressing the reproductive history of the various cohorts, such as mean number of children, mean age at the first childbirth, or other similar indicators. Naming such a factor f, we can define an age, period, and fertility model:

$$\textit{log } I \text{ or } \textit{logit } I = \Theta_o + \sum_i \Theta_{1i}\, x^i + \sum_j \Theta_{2j}\, y^j + \Theta_4\, f\,. \tag{9}$$

As a second example, consider the data on smoking history collected by a survey of a representative sample of the population. The information about the proportion of smokers, the mean age of starting, the mean number of cigarettes smoked, and the mean age of stopping allows one to estimate theoretically the past exposure of each generation at each point in time. Let s be the variable expressing exposure. It varies in time within a generation and therefore can be added to the age, period, and cohort model:

$$\textit{log } I \text{ or } \textit{logit } I = \Theta_o + \sum_i \Theta_{1i}\, x^i + \sum_j \Theta_{2j}\, y^j + \sum_k \Theta_{3k}\, z^k + \Theta_5\, s\,. \tag{10}$$

In this section, some examples of morbidity models have been described. The functions (7)-(10) are flexible enough to represent complex incidence patterns with a relatively small number of parameters. Many different functions can of course be constructed; in particular, cross-product terms can be added if the hypothesis that each factor carries an independent multiplicative contribution to the risk of the disease is to be disregarded.

Application: Estimating Cancer Morbidity in Italy

Estimates of incidence and prevalence for various diseases - total cancer [8, 9], myocardial infarction [10], breast cancer [11], and stomach cancer [6] - have been carried out in Italy from mortality data. The most relevant results for all cancers in the male population were as follows:

Mortality and population data for the years 1960-83, by single-year age classes, were used for estimation procedures. It was rather difficult to obtain survival data, since no reliable estimates were available on the survival of cancer patients in Italy. The main source of these data was the curves observed in the USA and described by the SEER program publications [12, 13]. The reported survival curves were initially adjusted by cancer site distribution, which differ between the USA and Italy. A proportional hazard assumption was then made to model the age dependency of survival rates, and the values of the age parameters were estimated from the SEER age-specific survival curves.

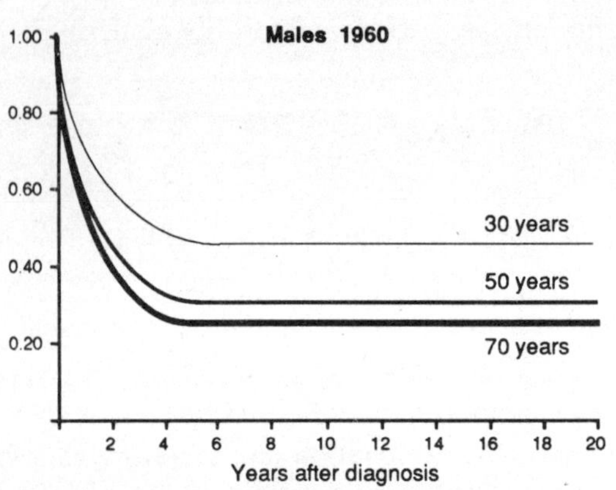

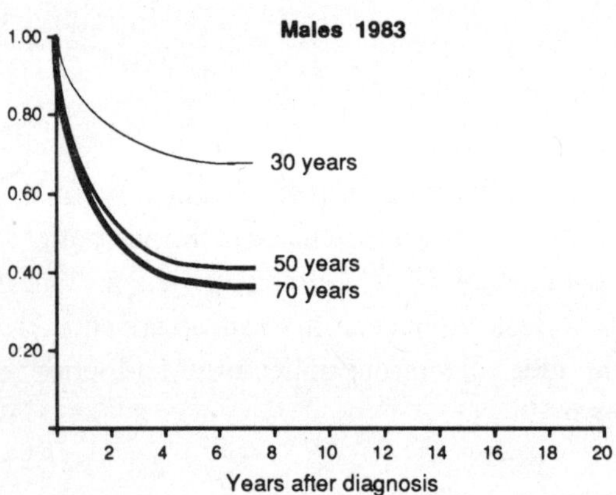

Fig. 2. Relative survival of male cancer patients at selected ages, by year of diagnosis

The relative survival curves thereby obtained for the first and the last year of the period considered are shown in Figure 2, for selected ages. For the intervening years, the values were estimated by a linear interpolation between the two extremes for each age of diagnosis. Details of the calculation of survival curves are reported in reference [8].

For a first example of application we ignore the age dependency of survival, and accept all assumptions leading to the reduced equation system (2). We then consider survival rates for cancer patients of all ages in a single year (say, in 1983), and try to fit the observed values with an exponential function defined by the death density (3). The obtained parameter values are $A = 0.634$, $\lambda = 0.89$. It is then easy to obtain from expression (4) simple estimates of age-specific incidence rates in the considered year. The scheme of the calculation is shown in Table 1. The first two columns indicate the years of birth of the generations being considered and

Table 1. Scheme for the calculation of age-specific incidence rates from expression (4). Italy, male population

Birth cohort	Age in 1983	Mortality · 10 000 1982	1983	1984	$\frac{dM}{dx}$	Incidence estimated in 1983
1948-1953	30-34	1.7	1.7	2.0	0.15	2.9
1943-1948	35-39	3.2	3.3	3.9	0.35	5.8
1938-1943	40-44	6.4	7.6	8.5	1.05	13.8
1933-1938	45-49	13.1	15.0	16.5	1.70	26.6
1928-1933	50-54	26.4	30.9	32.5	3.05	54.1
1923-1928	55-59	46.5	52.2	55.6	4.05	90.5
1918-1923	60-64	70.0	78.2	83.5	7.75	137.1
1913-1918	65-69	103.1	111.9	119.3	8.10	190.9
1908-1913	70-74	139.5	147.3	154.6	7.55	245.7

their ages in the year 1983. Columns 3-5 report the mortality rates of each cohort in the years 1982, 1983, and 1984. Column 6 gives an estimate of expression (4). This quantity is computed by dividing by two the difference between the mortality rates of the cohort in 1984 and 1982. Finally, the last column reports the estimated age-specific incidence rates.

This is, of course, a sample application of mainly illustrative value. The estimated incidence rates are to be considered as quick and rough approximations, since they are based upon a number of assumptions not fully verified in the particular case being considered. It is nonetheless interesting to compare these rates with the corresponding values obtained from a more rigorous estimation procedure, taking particular account of the age and time variability of survival rates.

Statistical estimations of morbidity function parameters were then carried out, using the system equation (1) to link a logistic age, period, and cohort incidence model (8) to the observed mortality data in the years 1960 to 1983. An incidence function of order 3 for age, of order 2 for period, and finally of order 3 for cohort resulted from the stepwise procedure. The observed age-specific and standardized mortality rates, and the estimated incidence rates and prevalence for the years 1960 and 1983 are presented in Table 2.

Table 2. Cancer mortality and estimated morbidity in Italian male population. Age-specific and standardized rates, prevalence (· 10 000), and corresponding percent annual change in the period 1960-1983. Incidence and prevalence are estimated by the age, period, and cohort model (8)

	Mortality			Incidence			Prevalence		
Age	1960	1983	% annual change	1960	1983	% annual change	1960	1983	% annual change
30-34	2.2	1.7	-1.12	4.6	5.9	1.08	22	41	2.7
35-39	3.7	3.3	-0.50	7.5	10.1	1.29	32	60	2.8
40-44	6.8	7.6	0.48	12.9	17.4	1.30	49	91	2.7
45-49	12.9	15.0	0.66	21.5	31.0	1.59	73	139	2.8
50-54	23.6	30.9	1.17	36.9	53.4	1.61	111	212	2.8
55-59	40.3	52.2	1.12	59.5	88.6	1.73	169	329	2.9
60-64	61.1	78.2	1.07	90.6	142.2	1.97	248	497	3.0
65-69	83.2	111.9	1.29	124.5	190.2	1.84	353	769	3.4
70-74	102.7	147.3	1.57	154.3	251.4	2.12	423	931	3.4
stand.	26.3	34.1	1.13	40.5	61.4	1.81	120	244	3.0

Outside the age range 30-74 years, mortality rates are either too low, or insufficiently reliable with regard to identifying the cause of death. Results were thus reported only for this age range.

The same results have been extensively presented and discussed elsewhere [9]. Due to the mainly illustrative purpose of this application, only the most relevant points will be discussed here. In particular, it can be seen that:

- incidence increases with age less than mortality (the mortality/incidence ratio in the year 1983 rises from 0.29 in the first age class to 0.59 in the last one);
- incidence increases with age more than prevalence (about 6 prevalent cases are estimated in the same year for each incident case in the youngest ages, as compared to 4 in the oldest);
- the rate of incidence increase with age is fairly constant (about 1.7 each 5 years) until 65 years, and then decreases;
- within the period under consideration, we estimate almost a doubling of the standardized incidence rate, a three-fold increase of the prevalence, and an increase of only 13% in mortality;

- both incidence and prevalence show an increasing trend for all age classes, in contrast with mortality, which decreases for the youngest cohorts.

From a general point of view, the morbidity analysis presented here successfully used the available survival information in order to disentangle patterns of morbidity from those of mortality. The increase in survival rates within the considered period resulted in diverging incidence, prevalence, and mortality time trends. Age variability of survival led to different shapes of incidence, prevalence, and mortality age schedules.

A comparison of these results with those obtained by the simpler model (4), and reported in Table 1, indicates very similar values for ages over 50 years. This is not true for the youngest ages, where the incidence values computed by expression (4) are much lower than the corresponding values estimated by model (6). This is mainly due to the fact that the former estimates do not take into account the age variability of survival. When the overall survival is lower than the age-specific survival, expression (4) tends to underestimate incidence.

References

1. Klementiev AA (1977) On estimation of morbidity. IIASA, Laxenburg, pp 1-23
2. Kitsul P (1980) A dynamic approach to the estimation of morbidity. IIASA, Laxenburg, pp 1-25
3. Manton KG, Stallard E (1982) The use of mortality time series data to produce hypothetical morbidity distributions and project mortality trends. Demography 19:223-240
4. Verdecchia A, Capocaccia R, Mazzoni C (1985) Estimation of cancer morbidity using mortality data. Tumori 71:431-439
5. Verdecchia A, Capocaccia R, Egidi V, Golini A (1989) A method for the estimation of chronic disease morbidity and trends from mortality data. Statistics in Medicine 8:201-216
6. Capocaccia R Relationships between incidence and mortality in non-reversible disease. (Manuscript submitted for publication)
7. Frome EL (1983) The analysis of rates using Poisson regression models. Biometrics 39:665-674
8. Egidi V, Golini A, Capocaccia R, Verdecchia A (1988) Un model d'evaluation de l'etat de santé de la population a partir de mesures de la mortalité: le cas du cancer. In: Vallin J, D'Souza S, Palloni A (eds) Mesure et analyse de la mortalité. Nouvelles approches. INED and IUSSP, Travaux et Documents Cahier 119, Presses Universitaires de France, pp 425-442
9. Egidi V, Verdecchia A, Hanau C (1988) Cancer morbidity in Italy: an assessment of trends and influence on health care and the economy. (Paper presented at the XXIVth Conference of the Applied Econometrics Association on Demographic Modelling, Verona, Italy, February 1988)

10. Verdecchia A, Capocaccia R, Mazzoni C (1984) Estimation of cardiovascular diseases morbidity using mortality data. In: van Eimeren W, Engelbrecht R, Flagle CD (eds) Proceedings of the third international conference on system science and health care. Springer, Berlin Heidelberg New York, pp 44-47
11. Capocaccia R, Verdecchia A, Micheli A, Sant M, Gatta G, Berrino F (1990) Breast cancer incidence and prevalence estimated from survival and mortality. Cancer Causes and Control 1:23-29
12. Axtell LM (1976) Cancer patient survival. Report No. 5 NIH Publication No. 81, p 992
13. Ries LG, Pollack ES, Young JL (1983) Cancer patient survival: surveillance, epidemiology, and end results program 1973-79. J Nat Cancer Inst 70:693-707

A Probabilistic Model for Cancer Prevalence Estimation on Mortality Data

A. I. Michalski and A. I. Yashin

Basic Conceptions

The model is based on the assumption that any person in the population may be in one of three states: no cancer, cancer, terminal state. *No cancer* state means that a person in this state has good health or has any other disease except cancer. The state *cancer* means that a person in this state has cancer but it may be not diagnosed yet. This case we consider as a latent case of cancer because the disease process in this case is not observed. The transition from *no cancer* to *cancer* state corresponds to the cancer morbidity process.

We consider three different ways of transitions to the terminal state. The first way is the transition from *no cancer* state. This transition is related with causes of death different from cancer. We call the rate of this transition as *no cancer mortality. No cancer mortality* may be applied to transition from *cancer* state to the terminal one either. This is a case when a person with cancer dies from a cause different from cancer. This is the second way to get to the terminal state. The third way corresponds to the case when a person with cancer dies from cancer. The rate of this transition we call *personal cancer mortality.*

Let's make following assumptions about personal rates of transitions. We assume that *no cancer mortality* depends on the person's age and is the same for both *no cancer* and *cancer* states. This assumption means that cancer does not affect on a personal resistance to the other disease. It's not true for the real life but in the lack of information about the relation between cancer and the other diseases this rough assumption is valid. The *no cancer mortality* is to be extracted from the population data. The *personal cancer mortality* depends on a person's age and on the duration of the period the person remains in the *cancer* state. This mortality may be extracted from clinical studies. The personal rate of *no cancer* to *cancer* transition we consider to be unknown. It is the aim of this paper to describe a procedure for this rate estimation. The estimation of *no cancer* to *cancer* transition rate may be used for cancer prevalence estimation, estimation of the life expectancy in good health and the other important population characteristics.

The basic idea of the approach is that the transitions between the states has probabilistic nature. The cancer prevalence is a probability to be in the state *no*

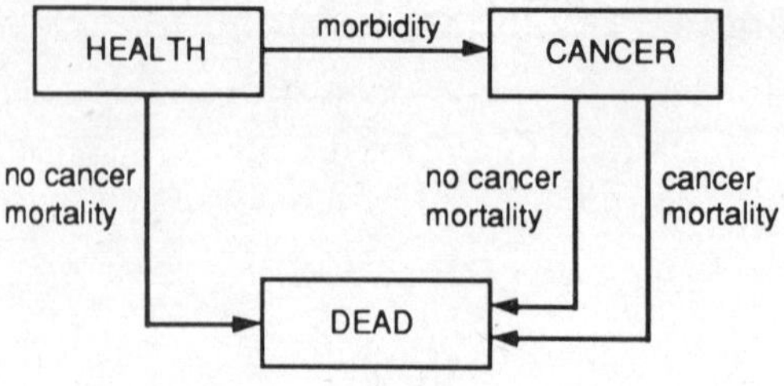

Fig.1. The structure of the PMCP model

cancer at specific age. The mean time which a person stays in *no cancer* state is the *health life expectancy*. The cancer morbidity is a rate of transition from *no cancer* to *cancer* states. This morbidity differs from registered cancer morbidity in population because it takes into account latent persons with cancer. Cancer mortality in population is related with latent cancer morbidity. This relation is used for calculations in Probabilistic Model for Cancer Prevalence – PMCP model. The structure of the model is given in Figure 1.

Mathematical Description

Let $\mu_1(x)$ be *no cancer mortality* rate, $\lambda(x)$ be the rate of *no cancer* to *cancer* state transition, $\mu_2(x)$ be the rate of death on cancer after suffering cancer during x years. Then the surviving function may be expressed in the form [1]

$$S(x) = e^{-\int_0^x \mu_1(\tau)\,d\tau} \left[1 - \int_0^x \left(1 - e^{-\int_{x-y}^{x} (\mu_1(\tau) + \mu_2(\tau))\,d\tau} \right) g(y)\,dy \right] \qquad (1)$$

where $g(y) = \lambda(y)\, e^{-\int_0^y \lambda(\tau)\,d\tau}$ is density function for probability of *no cancer* to *cancer* state transition. The expression (1) is an integral equation of Volterra type in relation to the function $g(y)$.

The solution of integral equation (1) may be calculated numerically but there is a problem of unstability. The unstability means that small disturbances in the survival function $S(x)$ may lead to big changes in the corresponding solution $g(y)$. This property may cause dramatic results if the survival function $S(x)$ is estimated on the base of population statistics. To stabilize the solution of the equation (1) we calculate it in the form of cubic spline-function. The parameters of the spline are calculated using least squares procedure. The number of spline's knots on the equidistant greed is the key question of this approach. The less the number of the knots is the more stable the spline-solution of the equation (1) is. The more the number of spline's knots is the better the cubic spline approximates the real solution of the integral equation but the less stable the spline-solution is. This contradiction may be overcome by using an optimal number of spline's knots or by selecting an optimal model for equation (1) solution. We put description of the procedure for the optimal model selection in the appendix.

The probability to be at age x in the state *cancer* may be expressed in the form

$$P_2(x) = e^{-\int_0^x \mu_1(\tau)\,d\tau} \int_0^x e^{-\int_{x-y}^{x} (\mu_1(\tau) + \mu_2(t))\,d\tau}\, g(y)\,dy \;. \qquad (2)$$

The mathematical expectation of *good health* life span is calculated by the formula

$$T_h = \int_0^\infty e^{-\int_0^x \mu_1(\tau)\,d\tau} \left(1 - \int_0^x g(y)\,dy \right) dx \,. \qquad (3)$$

Results of Calculations

PMCP model was used for estimation of male cancer prevalence in Japan for two years: 1947 and 1972. The calculations were made for *general cancer* data. Total male mortality and cancer male mortality were extracted as functions of age from the sources available in the Population Program unit of the International Institute of Applied Systems Analysis (IIASA, Laxenburg, Austria). The surviving on *general cancer* state was used in exponential form with death rate, corresponding to life expectancy equal to five years. It is a rough estimation of surviving among persons with *general cancer* but nevertheless some interesting results were obtained.

The results of calculations are as follows: for both years -1947 and 1972- the optimal number of knots in the spline-solution of equation (1) was selected to be equal to 1. On the base of spline-solution the probability to be at age x in the state *general cancer* or cancer prevalence was calculated by the formula (2).

Table 1 shows the numbers of people in states *no cancer* and *cancer* at different ages. The numbers were estimated for synthetic cohorts of 100 000 per-

Table 1. Distribution of health status for two synthetic cohorts of 100 000 persons (estimated with data from Japan 1947, 1972)

	1947		1972	
Ages	Number of persons in *no cancer* state	Number of persons in *cancer* state	Number of persons in *no cancer* state	Number of persons in *cancer* state
0	100000	0	100000	0
5	89041	12	98818	39
10	87626	77	98574	36
15	86778	76	98374	27
20	84656	56	97842	28
25	80951	67	97205	46
30	77342	148	96508	83
35	74037	218	95675	144
40	70818	242	94445	237
45	67292	287	92598	398
50	62898	505	89986	722
55	57092	872	86040	1259
60	49442	1209	80089	1961
65	39874	1201	71246	2804
70	29157	901	59013	3353
75	18577	515	43836	3186
80	9787	202	27570	2129
≥85	3972	53	13287	925

sons on the base of mortality data for Japan males in 1947 and 1972 using formulas (1) and (2). One can see that the portion of people in the state *cancer* in 1972 exceeds the same portion for 1947.

Table 2 shows the dynamic of cancer morbidity processes in 1947 and 1972. There are durations of *no cancer* life span at different ages. The values were estimated on the base of mortality data for Japan males in 1947 and 1972 using formula (3). The life expectancies at different ages were put in the table. From the table one can see that for all ages the life expectancy in 1972 increased in comparison with the life expectancy in 1947. But at the same time almost for all ages the proportion of the *no cancer* span in the life expectancy decreased for 1972 in comparison with 1947. The last means that year 1972 gained more life expectancy from year 1947 but the *quality* of this gain was poore. There are many possible explanations of this effect. It may be a result of elimination of

Table 2. Life expectancy and *cancer-free* life expectancy for two synthetic cohorts (estimated with data from Japan 1947 and 1972)

	Life expectancy		*Cancer free* life expectancy		% of life expectancy free of cancer	
Ages	1947	1972	1947	1972	1947	1972
0	52.19	70.50	51.86	69.62	99.36	98.75
5	53.43	66.30	53.07	65.44	99.32	98.70
10	49.22	61.46	48.89	60.60	99.32	98.60
15	44.68	56.58	44.34	55.71	99.23	98.46
20	40.73	51.87	40.38	51.00	99.14	98.32
25	37.47	47.19	37.11	46.32	99.03	98.15
30	34.07	42.49	33.73	41.64	99.00	97.99
35	30.45	37.82	30.12	36.98	98.91	97.77
40	26.70	33.24	26.38	32.42	98.80	97.53
45	22.95	28.79	22.63	28.02	98.60	97.32
50	19.29	24.45	19.02	23.75	98.60	97.13
55	15.85	20.30	15.69	19.72	98.99	97.14
60	12.76	16.43	12.72	15.99	99.68	97.32
65	10.14	12.92	10.12	12.64	99.80	97.83
70	7.93	9.85	7.91	9.72	99.74	98.68
75	6.06	7.22	6.05	7.21	99.83	99.86
80	4.42	4.97	4.41	4.96	99.77	99.79
≥85	2.62	2.79	2.61	2.78	99.61	99.64

some causes of death in Japan in 1972 in comparison with 1949 or it may be the effect of air and food pollution and so on. It is a matter of further investigations to make more precise estimations and to find main risk factors in connection with cancer mortality.

Appendix

In this appendix we describe a procedure for a model selection on the base of empirical data. The idea of the procedure is to select in the given set of algorithms π the *best* algorithm. The *best* algorithm produces the *best* model. We will show that for the specific case of modelling using least squares procedure the *best* algorithm is to minimize a criterion:

$$k_n = \frac{J_n}{\frac{m - 2n}{m}}$$

where m is the number of observations, n is the number of parameters in the model and J_n is the value of square residuals for least squares procedure. Considering models with different numbers of parameters we choose the optimal model.

Let's denote $T = \{x_1, y_1, \ldots\ldots, x_m, y_m\}$ a set of random variables which are connected by the relationship

$$y_j = f(x_j) + \varepsilon_j \qquad j = 1, \ldots\ldots, m \tag{a.1}$$

where $f(\cdot)$ is an unknown deterministic function, ε_j is an independent random variable with $M(\varepsilon_j) = 0$ and $D(\varepsilon_j) = \sigma_j^2$. The general problem is: *how to estimate function $f(\cdot)$ on the base of sample T?*

The relationship (a.1) describes different practical situations. It may be used if values of observed function $f(x)$ are disturbed by some *noise*. Then on the base of sample T one estimates undisturbed values of function $f(x)$. The other case of interest is related with dependent pair of random variables {X,Y}. In this case the sample T is the set of this pair realizations, function $f(x)$ is the function of conditional mathematical expectation and one is to estimate the function of conditional mathematical expectation on the base of sample T. The third case is the case of operator relation. In this case function $f(x)$ may be the result of some other function $g(t)$ transformation. The transformation may be in the form of an integral operator.

$$f(x) = \int_a^b K(x,t)\, g(t)\, dt$$

where $K(x,t)$ is the *kernel function*, [a,b] is the interval of $g(t)$ function definition. In the case of operator relation one is to estimate the solution of operator equation on the base of sample T. The specific case of integral equation is equation of Volterra type

$$f(x) = \int_a^x K(x,t)\, g(t)\, dt \ . \tag{a.2}$$

The equation of this type describes the surviving process in the probabilistic model for cancer prevalence [1] which was described in the main text of this article.

To select an algorithm for equation solution we consider a set of algorithms π which estimates this solution on the base of random sample T. It may be, for example, a set of operators that construct an estimate of function g(t) by the least squares procedure in the form of algebraic polynomials of different degrees or in the form of cubic spline functions with different numbers of knots. We will find the performance for every algorithms ***A*** from the set π when using sample T in the next part of this appendix. We denote this performance by $G(\boldsymbol{A})$. The performance will not depend on the unknown function g(t) but it will depend on the algorithm ***A*** and the sample T. To find the best estimate we are to find in the set π the algorithm with the best performance $G(\boldsymbol{A})$ and use it to estimate the solution of the equation (a.2).

Let us denote by P(x,y) the joint distribution function of random variables X and Y according to which the sample of independent pairs (x_i, y_i), $T = \{x_1, y_1, \ldots\ldots, x_m, y_m\}$ has been generated. Let g(t) be an estimate of integral equation (a.2) solution. We define the performance of the estimate g(t) and the performance of an algorithm ***A*** which was used to obtain the estimate g(x).

The performance of the fixed function g(t) may be determined as the average risk functional defined by the formula

$$I(g) = \int \left(y - \int_a^b K(x,t)\, g(t)\, dt\right)^2 dP(x,y) \ .$$

It is easy to see that the minimal value of the functional $I(g)$ is reaching on the function on the solution of the integral equation.

Let a function g(t) be a result of calculations by an algorithm ***A*** on the sample T. In this case g(t) is a random function and the functional $I(g)$ is a random variable. Denote the performance of the algorithm ***A*** as the average value of the functional $I(g)$. The averaging is to be made on all samples of independent random pairs (x_i, y_i) with the joint distribution function P(x, y). The formula for the algorithm ***A*** performance is

$$G(\boldsymbol{A}) = \int I(g)\, dP(x_1, y_1, \ldots\ldots, x_m, y_m) \ .$$

The problem is how to calculate the functional $G(\boldsymbol{A})$ when the joint distribution function P(x, y) is not known. We will give the estimate for $G(\boldsymbol{A})$ in a case of linear estimating algorithms. Let $\hat{f}(x)$ be an estimate of the function $f(x)$ calculated by an algorithm ***A*** on the sample T. Denote $\hat{f}_i$ the value of function $\hat{f}(x)$ in the point x_i, i.e. $\hat{f}_i = \hat{f}(x_i)$. If ***A*** is a linear algorithm then the next relation is valid

$$\mathrm{F} = \boldsymbol{A}\,\mathrm{Y}$$

where $F = (\hat{f}_1, \ldots\ldots, \hat{f}_m)^T$, $Y = (y_1, \ldots., y_m)^T$ are vectors, $\mathbf{A}$ is a (m x m) – dimensional estimation matrix that corresponds to the linear algorithm. To estimate functional $G(\boldsymbol{A})$ we consider the expression for the empirical risk functional $J_e(\boldsymbol{A})$

$$J_e(\boldsymbol{A}) = \frac{\sum_{i=1}^{m}(y_i - \hat{f}_i)^2}{m} = \frac{\| F - Y \|^2}{m} = \frac{\| (\mathbf{E} - \mathbf{A}) Y \|^2}{m}$$

where $\mathbf{E}$ is the identity matrix. It is shown in [1] that for a fixed matrix $\mathbf{A}$

$$G(\boldsymbol{A}) = MJ_e(\boldsymbol{A}) - \frac{\sigma^2 \operatorname{Tr}(\mathbf{E} - 2\mathbf{A})}{m} + \sigma^2 . \tag{a.3}$$

The expression (a.3) contains the unknown mean value of empirical risk $MJ_e(\boldsymbol{A})$. This value is easy to estimate if algorithm $\boldsymbol{A}$ is fixed. In the case of algorithm selection we must construct a uniform estimate in the set of algorithms π. Such uniform estimate is constructed for linear algorithms set in [2]. We skip mathematical details and give the main result.

The result is as follows: if

- the value $M\varepsilon_j^4$ is finite, where ε_j is the random variable from the relation (a.1), $\sigma_j^2 \le \sigma_j$;
- the set π is composed from the linear algorithms based on the least squares procedure,

then with the probability no less than $1 - \eta$ the inequality is valid

$$\sup_{\boldsymbol{A} \in \pi} | MJ_e(\boldsymbol{A}) - J_e(\boldsymbol{A}) | \le \frac{B}{\sqrt{m\eta}} \tag{a.4}$$

where B is a constant value depending on moments of the random variable ε_j and properties of the set π.

The value of functional $G(\boldsymbol{A})$ now may be estimated using (a.4) by the expression

$$G(\boldsymbol{A}) = J_e(\boldsymbol{A}) + \frac{\sigma^2 \operatorname{Tr}(\mathbf{E} - 2\mathbf{A})}{m} + \sigma^2 + \frac{B}{\sqrt{m\eta}}$$

which is valid with the probability no less than $1 - \eta$.

In the right-hand side of the last inequality only the first two terms depend on the algorithm $\boldsymbol{A}$. It means that the sum of these two terms may be used as a criterion for selection of the best algorithm in the set π

$$C(\boldsymbol{A}) = J_e(\boldsymbol{A}) + \frac{\sigma^2 \, \mathrm{Tr}\,(\mathbf{E} - 2\boldsymbol{A})}{m}. \tag{a.5}$$

The expression (a.5) may be used if the value of noise variance σ^2 is known. To construct a criterion for the case of unknown σ^2 we rewrite the expression (a.5) in form

$$C(\boldsymbol{A}) = \frac{m - 2\mathrm{Tr}\mathbf{A}}{m} \left(\frac{m J_e(\boldsymbol{A})}{m - 2\mathrm{Tr}\mathbf{A}} - \sigma^2 \right).$$

By confining ourselves to the case $0 < 2\mathrm{Tr}\mathbf{A}$, we obtain an inequality

$$C(\boldsymbol{A}) < \frac{J_e(\boldsymbol{A})}{\frac{m - 2\mathrm{TrA}}{m}}$$

whose right-hand side may be taken as a criterion of selection of an algorithm from the class π that does not depend on the noise variance. We denote the criterion K($\boldsymbol{A}$) and will call it *statistical elimination criterion*

$$K(\boldsymbol{A}) = \frac{J_e(\boldsymbol{A})}{\frac{m - 2\mathrm{Tr}\boldsymbol{A}}{m}}. \tag{a.6}$$

The criterion K($\boldsymbol{A}$) takes simple form if the set π contains algorithms based on the least squares procedure in the subspaces of different finite dimensions. For this case Tr$\mathbf{A}$ = n where n is the dimension of the subspace in which the algorithm $\boldsymbol{A}$ is defined. The *statistical elimination criterion* takes the form

$$K_n(\boldsymbol{A}) = \frac{J_n(\boldsymbol{A})}{\frac{m - 2n}{m}}.$$

References

1. Michalski AI, Petrovski AM, Yashin AI (1989) The theory of estimation in heterogeneous populations. Nauka, Moscow, p 127
2. Michalski AI (1987) Choosing an algorithm of estimation based on samples of limited size. Automation and Remote Control 36 (7):57-66

PREVENT, a Model to Estimate the Health Benefits of Prevention

L. J. Gunning-Schepers, J. J. M. Barendregt and P. J. van der Maas

Introduction

In health policy making, there has been a shift in recent years away from the pure planning of health services towards a comprehensive health planning, in which an attempt is made to use increasingly scarce resources in such a way as to achieve *maximal* health for the population. This shift is exemplified by the WHO campaign *Health for All by the year 2000,* and by the use of targets in the European region [1]. This shift has two interesting features. One is a tendency to measure the effectiveness of a policy, intervention or technology in terms of health as the outcome, rather than in terms of the input, output, or process. The other is an acceptance that choices need to be made since, however large the budget for health, it will always be limited. Most of the attention given to this last concern in recent years has been political, but both features have generated a demand for a different kind of information on which to base policy decisions. The orientation towards health has spurred an interest in the health benefits to be expected from interventions, at both the individual and the population level. Concern with the optimization of scarce resources has led to a keen interest in cost-effectiveness, both for the individual patient and for policy making at the population level.

One question which is much debated in health planning is the amount to be invested in primary prevention. Acknowledging that health is also influenced by the prevalence of risk factors in a population, and not only by health care, comprehensive health planning will have to weigh investments in primary prevention against investments in curative services. Investments in prevention are not as popular as they used to be. Contrary to curative care, where decisions are taken in the doctor's office, usually between two consenting adults, decisions on collective prevention are most often taken in the cumbersome bureaucracies that guard democracy. Increasingly in health planning, questions are being asked about the estimated rate of return on investment. For prevention, the prospects have not been good lately.

In the competition for limited resources, advocates of preventive interventions have had to support their claims with facts about the expected returns on such an investment. They have to explain that prevention now will not lead to visible health benefits tomorrow, but will at best result in the non-occurrence of a specific disease in the distant future. They have to do so, moreover, at a time when the major multifactorial intervention trials are yielding disappointing results and new curative technologies are being widely acclaimed. Some of the disappointment may be due to unrealistic expectations of the interventions, and to limitations in the methodology used to estimate the effects of prevention. If prevention is to compete for the allocation of scarce resources, it must be able to apply existing knowledge about risk factors to estimate realistically the health benefits to be expected from an intervention in these risk factors. Although epidemiology has been good at identifying the risk factors in which to intervene, the application of this epidemiological knowledge to health policy making is still primitive.

PREVENT, Applied Epidemiology

In The Netherlands, the PREVENT model was developed to help apply existing epidemiological knowledge to decision-making in health policy [2]. It is a simulation model that can estimate the health benefits for a population of changes in risk factor prevalence, both in terms of proportional changes in disease-specific incidence and in terms of absolute changes in, among other parameters, disease-specific and total mortality. The goal of the PREVENT project was to devise a tool for policy makers to use epidemiological data on the relationship between risk factors and diseases in order to estimate the effect on the health of a population of changes, either autonomous or through interventions, in risk factor prevalence. The type of information it provides can be useful in quantifying different lifestyle scenarios, exploring the different interventions necessary to achieve targets in health planning, or estimating the effects of alternative preventive interventions as input for more formal decision-making processes, such as cost-effectiveness analysis.

PREVENT uses epidemiology, but because the policy making perspective is somewhat different its application of epidemiology has generated some new areas of interest:

- Traditional epidemiology is mostly concerned with the increased incidence associated with exposure to a risk factor, whereas policy makers are more interested in the reduction of risk after the cessation of exposure. This risk reduction may take many years to achieve, so that estimates of effect will have to incorporate a time dimension.
- In traditional epidemiology, several risk factors are often identified for one disease. For preventive interventions, it is much more interesting when one

risk factor seems to affect several diseases. To estimate the potential effect of an intervention on a risk factor, all of these diseases should be considered.

- For policy making, it is not sufficient to look at carefully selected experimental populations. Results should be applicable to a real population, with all the dynamics inherent in such a population.

The PREVENT model attempts to incorporate these aspects in traditional epidemiological measures of effect, in order to serve as a tool for policy making.

Existing Epidemiological Measures in PREVENT

In epidemiology, analysis of the distribution of disease incidence and risk factor prevalence in different populations is used to confirm the hypothesis of a causal relationship between risk factor and disease. The strength of the relationship is often expressed as the ratio of incidence between exposed and non-exposed, the Incidence Density Ratio (IDR) or relative risk. The importance of a risk factor for the incidence of a disease in a population is usually expressed as the Etiologic Fraction (EF), the proportion of the total incidence of the disease that can be attributed to that risk factor in the population. This indicates the proportion of incidence that could be prevented by the total elimination of that risk factor in the population.

However, since prevention will usually not eliminate but merely reduce the prevalence of a risk factor, a measure was developed to estimate the impact of a change in prevalence of a risk factor on the incidence of a disease, the Potential Impact Fraction (PIF) [3]. It indicates the incidence that is avoided by a preventive intervention as a proportion of the incidence that would have occurred in that population without the intervention. Both the EF and the PIF can be calculated when P's, the prevalences of exposure to a risk factor in the population, and the corresponding IDR's are known. The potential impact fraction in the traditional epidemiological literature assumes an immediate elimination of excess risk after the termination of exposure. Those no longer exposed are returned to the category of non-exposed with, by definition, an IDR of 1.

The PREVENT Methodology

PREVENT's methodology is based on the epidemiological effect measure, PIF. To achieve the objectives stated, the following three requirements are included in the methodology:

- a time dimension, to simulate the reduction in excess risk after cessation of exposure to the risk factor;
- the possibility that one risk factor affects several diseases, and that one disease is affected by several risk factors;
- the interaction between the effect of the intervention and the demographic evolution of the population.

In the current version of PREVENT, all measures of health benefit are based on mortality. There are two steps in the methodology: in the first, PIFs are calculated, and in the second, these proportional measures are expressed as absolute health benefits. The first two requirements of the methodology are incorporated in the first step of the model, the third one dictated the format of the second step.

In the first step of the PREVENT model, several risk factors and several diseases are analyzed simultaneously. The prevalence of each risk factor is denoted by P, the proportion of the population or sub-population exposed in a certain exposure category. In order to use information on the causal relationship between risk factor exposure and disease incidence as effectively as possible, the prevalence is stratified by age and sex category. Since one risk factor can affect several diseases, each exposure category is assigned several IDRs, each representing the strength of the relationship between the risk factor and one of the diseases. Knowing the existing distribution of a population over exposure categories (P) and the corresponding IDRs, we can estimate the proportional changes in incidence (PIF) for each disease affected by that risk factor, due to changes in P, for example as a result of a preventive intervention. In a second step of the model these disease-specific PIFs are applied to the disease-specific mortality quotients and then to a population, so that the proportional PIFs are translated into absolute measures of health benefit.

An important element in the methodology was the introduction of a time dimension. For each risk factor and disease combination a time period in years is assumed between the moment of cessation of exposure and the moment the lowest relative risk for ex-exposed, the remnant IDR, is reached. This time period is called LAG. The introduction of this time dimension necessitates an adjustment of the equation used for the calculation of PIF, as well as an additional dimension of the input data on prevalence and IDR. It means that the ultimate PIF is not reached immediately after the intervention, but only after LAG years. It may take years before the intervention has its maximum effect. The time dimension also means however, that past changes in risk factor prevalence, whatever their cause, may continue to affect disease incidence in the future. This change in disease-specific incidence should not be ascribed to the intervention. To incorporate the proportional effect of such past (and possibly also future) *autonomous trends* in risk factor prevalences, PREVENT calculates Trend Impact Fractions (TIFs) in a manner similar to the PIFs.

By the end of LAG years the maximum PIF is reached; this is the effect of the intervention in proportional terms. The effect in absolute numbers, the health benefit, also depends on three other factors: (a) the proportional changes in disease-specific incidence over that same period caused by autonomous trend (the TIFs), (b) the relative contribution of the diseases, influenced by that specific risk factor, on total mortality, and (c) the demographic changes in the population over those LAG years. It is the time dimension in the first step of the model, and the fact that it may vary for different diseases, which makes the interaction between the PIFs and the demographic changes interesting. The second step of the model consists of a population model in one year age-groups to which disease-specific mortality quotients (M) are applied, to simulate the evolution of the population over time. The assumption is that the proportional changes in incidence from the first part of the model, the PIFs and TIFs, are translated into the same proportional changes in disease-specific mortality after a certain latency period, LAT.

If the TIFs only are applied, the resulting new disease-specific mortality quotients, and the evolution of the population, represent the so-called reference or trend scenario, the developments expected when no intervention takes place. If, however, both TIFs and PIFs are applied to the mortality quotients, the population evolves as would be expected as a result of the intervention. Note that prevalence changes in one risk factor may generate changes in disease-specific mortality quotients for several diseases, and that risk factors for which no intervention is simulated nevertheless may cause changes in mortality quotients through TIFs as a result of autonomous trends in risk factor prevalences. The differences between the reference and intervention populations represent the effect of the intervention, and can be expressed as several measures of health benefit: differences in mortality, potential years of life gained, etc. To see the full effect of an intervention on such a measure of health benefit, the model should simulate for at least LAG+LAT years.

A simplified version of the model is shown in Figure 1.

The PREVENT Model

The stratification, and the time dimensions necessary for the methodology, make it imperative that the calculations of health benefits be done on a computer simulation model. One objective of the project was that the tool developed should be useful for policy makers. We decided, at the outset, that it should be an interactive model which could run on an IBM-compatible micro-computer,

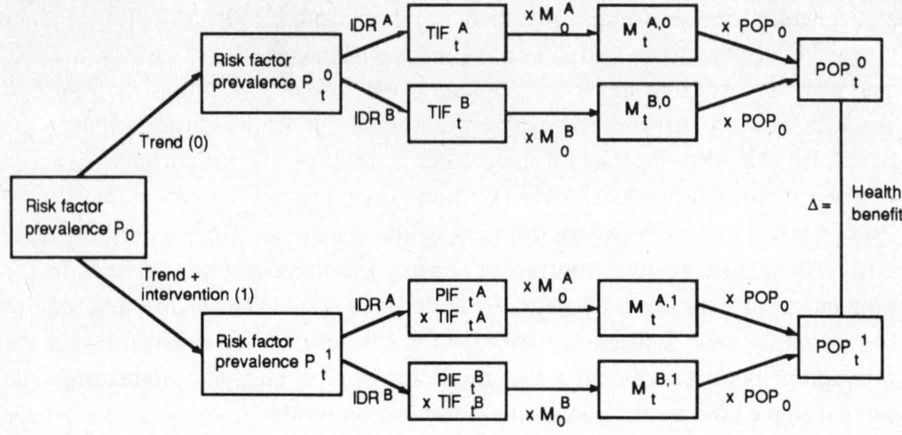

Fig. 1. The basic version of the PREVENT model

and which could be operated without prior knowledge of the epidemiological techniques used in the model.

The files containing the array of data on P and IDRs, the time dimensions, and the existing mortality quotients, and the population data can be adjusted for any population. In the first version of the model, the data were those for the Dutch population. In the current version, it is possible to create a different data base. This enables the model to be used for other populations, or even for other risk factors than the ones chosen in the original version.

For a simulation, the user can specify changes in risk factor prevalence as a result of autonomous trends or interventions, the time period over which the intervention occurs, the length of the simulation period, and whether the first, proportional part of the model will take a cohort factor into account. PREVENT will present the results in graphic or tabular form, for the intermediate output variables of EF, TIF, and PIF, and for the following outcome variables: disease-specific mortality, total mortality, (disease-specific) mortality difference, potential years of life gained, actual years of life gained, survival curves, and life expectancy at birth.

Results

In this section we show some results of typical PREVENT simulation runs. The examples have been chosen to illustrate the effect of the new elements added to the traditional epidemiological measures in the model. Since the model can be used directly by a policy maker, different interventions on the same risk factor can be compared before choosing the most desirable one.

A Time Dimension

In the first example, an intervention on the prevalence of cigarette smoking in the population is simulated. It is assumed that, without the intervention, there would be a continuing steady decrease in the number of smokers by 1% per year. The intervention consists of an abrupt 50% reduction in the number of smokers in all age, sex, and exposure categories in 1985.

Figure 2 shows the development of yearly lung cancer mortality in absolute numbers. The trend population shows the expected mortality if no intervention on smoking is made. The initial dip in male mortality is the result of the substantial reduction in the prevalence of smoking over the past ten years. Because of the time dimension, this reduction will continue to affect lung cancer mortality in the future. The subsequent steady increase reflects the rapid aging which will occur in the Dutch population in the years to come. The latency period between changes in incidence and changes in mortality explains why, in the first four years after intervention, no difference in lung cancer mortality between the trend and intervention populations is seen. There is then a slow reduction in lung cancer mortality in the intervention population, as the excess risk slowly diminishes after cessation of exposure. The difference in the evolution of both mortality curves shows the mortality reduction due to intervention. To appreciate the full benefit of this intervention, one should simulate for at least 15 years after the end of the intervention. This longer simulation also shows that the reduction in mortality persists even after that time, as the effect far outlasts the intervention period.

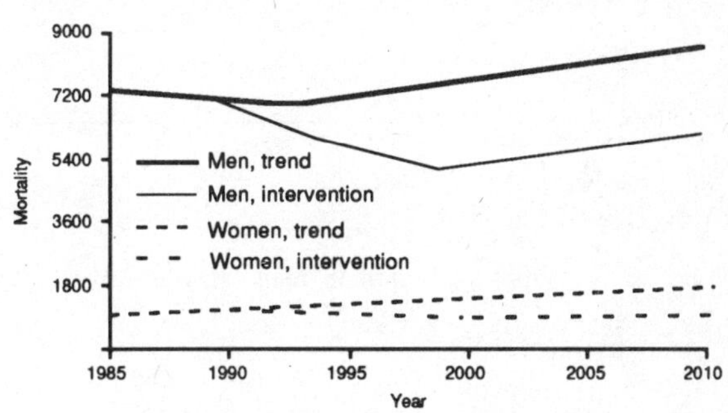

Fig. 2. Lung cancer mortality for men and women (absolute numbers), with and without intervention on smoking

A Multifactorial Model

The above intervention results not only in a reduction of lung cancer mortality. In the PREVENT model, cigarette smoking also affects Ischaemic Heart Disease (IHD) and Chronic Obstructive Lung Disease (COLD). One should, therefore, measure the health benefits not only in terms of a reduction in lung cancer mortality, but also as a reduction in total mortality.

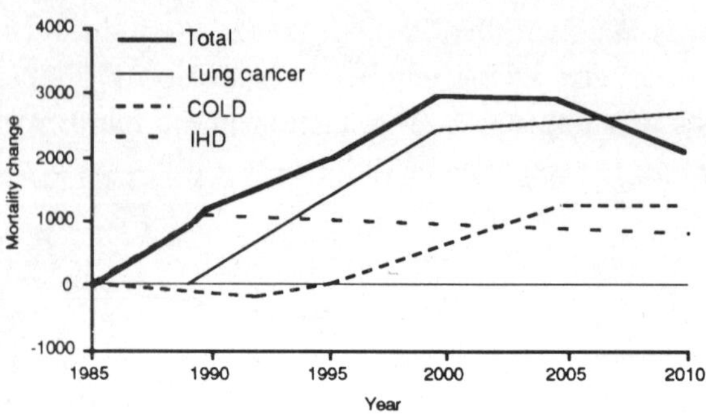

Fig. 3. Mortality reduction in men (absolute numbers) after an intervention on smoking

Figure 3 shows the total mortality reduction, in men, resulting from the intervention described above, as well as the mortality reduction in each individual disease category. The evolution of the total mortality curve clearly shows how each disease has its own time dimensions, and contributes to the mortality reduction at different points in time after the intervention. As it is apparent from Figure 2, a disease-specific mortality reduction is more or less constant once it has reached its maximum. But the total mortality reduction will eventually diminish as competing causes of death become more important. The mortality reduction shown is the net mortality benefit in the intervention population each year.

If this smoking reduction were part of a programme to prevent IHD, and its benefits were compared, for example, with those of new curative possibilities, one can easily see how much these benefits would be underestimated if only one disease category were considered. In the year 2000, for example, the mortality reduction for IHD is only about one-third of the total mortality reduction. When estimating the effects of a preventive intervention, it is important to consider all its health effects, both the positive ones for those diseases directly linked to the risk factor of the intervention, and the negative effects of a possible increase in other causes of death. The above example shows how greatly the net benefit may be underestimated if only one disease category is considered.

A Non-Intervention Population

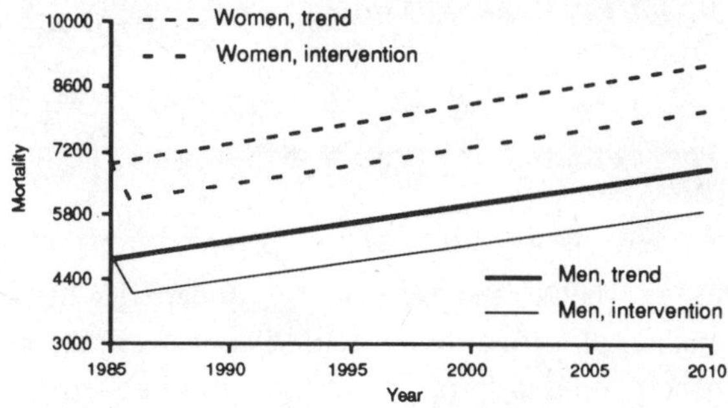

Fig. 4. CVA mortality in men and women (absolute numbers), with and without an intervention on hypertension

Figure 4 represents the mortality from CVA (Cerebrovascular accidents) after a hypothetical 50% reduction in hypertension in 1985 due to an intervention. It is clear that the unrealistically large shift in risk factor prevalence will not prevent the mortality (and thus the underlying number of cases) from exceeding the current number long before the year 2000. Has prevention then failed? No, but the demographic changes in this population will be considerable in the coming 15 years and the effect will be a steady rise in absolute CVA mortality. If no preventive intervention were applied, the mortality would be even higher in the year 2000.

This example is used only to illustrate why a trend population is essential when the effects of an intervention are assessed. Of course, one could present effect estimates as age-specific mortality rates and show that the preventive intervention leads to a sharp decrease. But policy makers have to work with a real population, and the impression should not be created that a reduction in age-specific mortality rates will always result in a net reduction in the number of real cases.

In an aging population with many chronic diseases in old age, a successful preventive intervention, causing a marked decline in the age-specific incidence rate, may still result in a higher number of cases in the population, as the age-group to which the reduced incidence rates apply increases in absolute numbers. This is often difficult to explain and makes it difficult to *sell* the intervention politically, since an appreciation of the health benefits requires an understanding of the dynamics underlying the effect estimates, and a visualization of what would occur in the absence of the intervention. In this example, the point is not that the effect estimates are different, but that results can be presented in such a way as to prevent unnecessary disappointment. One can also underestimate the effects of prevention, by not knowing what would have happened without the intervention.

PREVENT as a Tool

The Potential for Policy Making

To evaluate the utility of such a model in health policy making, it seems useful to see whether the expected health benefits are significantly changed by the inclusion of a time dimension, several diseases, and the possibility of expressing benefits in both proportional and absolute terms.

The time dimension is the PREVENT feature whose effect is most easily perceived. The long time lags between an intervention and observed changes in mortality from some diseases greatly affect the perceived results. The inclusion of a time dimension not only emphasizes that, in some cases, the results of preventive measures will not be noticeable immediately, but also shows that such a measure will continue to affect the population's health long after the intervention has ceased. To observe the expected effects over too short a period may lead to a serious underestimation of the ultimate benefits. The main interest in the multifactorial approach of the PREVENT model lies in the fact that not all diseases affect a health indicator (expressed in absolute numbers) to the same extent, and that the important time variables differ by disease. This means that a given risk factor intervention will reduce total mortality through several disease-specific mortalities, each to a different extent and at different times. This can be seen in the mortality reduction curve (Figure 3) of a reduction in smoking prevalence, in which the contribution of the different diseases can be clearly discerned.

It makes a difference whether the effects of an intervention are evaluated in a single-disease model or a multi-disease model. The multifactorial approach also dispels a commonly held belief: that competing death risks in our aging population will eliminate all mortality reduction from one disease, by substituting another cause of death. Although there is an increase in causes of death not affected by the risk factor intervened upon, nevertheless there is a large overall mortality reduction. When looking at the actual years of life gained by this intervention (Figure 5), one can conclude that the deaths prevented have indeed resulted in substantially extended lives. It is a fallacy to think that prevention will achieve an important mortality reduction only in a young population. Even in our aging population, we can achieve sizable mortality benefits.

The aggregation of health benefits and the introduction of a dynamic population, simulating the demographic evolution of the Dutch population, are essential to the second step of the model. When looking at disease-specific mortality, without intervention, it is obvious that demographic changes in the coming years will greatly increase absolute mortality for the diseases included

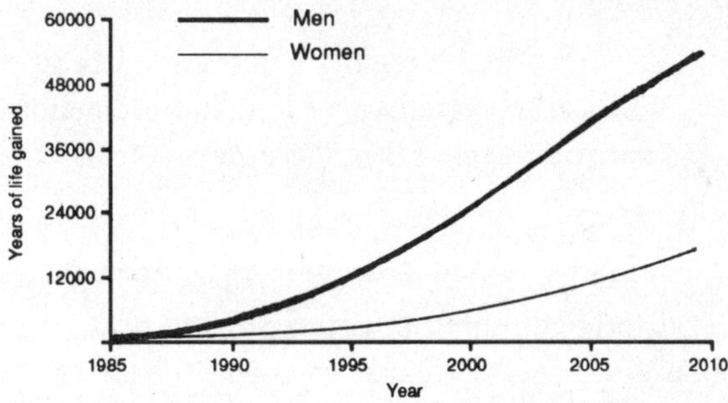

Fig. 5. Actual years of life (absolute numbers) gained after a smoking intervention

in PREVENT. In some cases, even far-reaching reductions in risk factor prevalence will not prevent the total number of cases from being higher in the future than they are today. In the Introduction, we stated that prevention is often difficult to *sell* politically since its effects take so long to become apparent. After the PREVENT exercise, we have to conclude that the situation is even worse: effects will seldom become apparent as real reductions in disease. This conclusion does not mean that prevention will have no beneficial effect in an aging population. On the contrary, it can result in a sizable mortality reduction despite competing death risks. It does mean, however, that in order to appreciate the effects, it is important to show what would happen without the preventive intervention, and not merely to compare them to the current level of mortality.

PREVENT at Work

Our efforts to make the model accessible to non-expert users have paid off. The model has been distributed nationally and internationally. Currently, it is being used in several places that we know of, mostly community health centres:

- In The Netherlands:
  - a number of community health services use it to determine priorities for their prevention policy, by ranking alternatives;.
  - it has been used as a teaching tool to visualize the health effects of interactions between changing mortality rates and demography, as well as cohort effects of risk factor prevalence;
  - it has been used as a tool to extrapolate the health effects of a regional risk factor intervention project in General Practice, to the national level.
- In Sweden,

  the Sundbyberg community health centres use the programme to monitor and evaluate their current prevention efforts.

- In Italy,

  in the Bergamo region, a prevention project is now being started which will use the programme to make projections of baseline disease-specific mortality, again for monitoring and evaluation.

- In Wales,

  it has been used to determine priorities in cancer policy.

Our original purpose was to provide a tool for policy makers. Looking back upon three years of experience with PREVENT's dissemination, we draw the following conclusions:

- In most cases, PREVENT was used with the Dutch data set to illustrate the possible health benefits of preventive interventions, since Western European populations are comparable in terms of risk factors and mortality patterns. In some cases, a local data set was introduced. Finding and preparing the input data in the necessary format proved more difficult than users had anticipated. Historical trends on risk factor prevalence data, and prevalence data that cover all age-groups, are not always routinely available.
- Interpreting the results of the model correctly continues to prove more complicated than we expected. Because of the interactions between risk factors, causes of death, and demography, basic epidemiological and demographic understanding are needed to be able to draw policy conclusions from the results.

In at least one instance, PREVENT was used incorrectly. We will elaborate here on this case because it is a good example of the risk of using such a model as a *black box*, without understanding the underlying dynamics.

In a report on the effects of fiscal reforms that are due in The Netherlands as a consequence of European economic unification, in particular the possible health effects of the harmonization of taxes on alcohol and tobacco [4], PREVENT was used to estimate the potential health benefits. On balance, this harmonization will result in higher taxes on cigarettes, and lower taxes on alcoholic beverages. A first, common-sense approach would suggest that, given normal (i.e. negative) price elasticities, the higher taxes on cigarettes would be beneficial for public health, and the lower taxes on alcohol detrimental. Not so, according to this report: both tax changes would lower mortality. So what happened? A closer look revealed a few minor mishaps, such as a misinterpretation of the model's output, and an attempt to calculate the effects of an increase in risk factor prevalence; the user is explicitly warned that the model is unsuitable for doing this.

But the main reason for the surprising result is use of the Ledermann hypothesis on the distribution of the consumption of alcohol in the population [5].

This hypothesis states:

- The consumption of alcohol can be described by a very skewed, lognormal distribution.
- There is a constant relationship between mean consumption and the prevalence of heavy drinking. In the present case, this was interpreted as a constant standard deviation.

The hypothesis is used as a convenient shorthand to estimate the number of excessive drinkers in a population: it is a lot easier to estimate the mean than the variance of consumption. Whatever the merits of the hypothesis, it is clearly meant to say something about the long thin tail of the distribution curve, but abstainers do not exist for the Ledermann model.

In PREVENT, abstainers do exist. The standard data set assumes, on epidemiological evidence, a U-shaped relationship between alcohol intake and risk of IHD, with moderate drinkers being the reference population, and abstainers and excessive drinkers having a relative risk of 2. Now, if one assumes a constant standard deviation while shifting the mean of the distribution, one will necessarily get a lower proportion of abstainers when the mean increases. And if the distribution is skewed enough, the proportion of abstainers turning into moderate drinkers will greatly outnumber the proportion of moderate drinkers becoming excessive drinkers. While this will indeed result in a higher mortality from cirrhosis, accidents, and IHD among excessive drinkers, this increase is swamped by the decrease in mortality from IHD due to the lower risk in abstainers who become moderate drinkers. So the reported health benefit of increased alcohol consumption comes from the highly improbable proposition that abstainers have the same price elasticity for alcohol as drinkers do. A completely inelastic demand of abstainers is surely closer to the truth.

This experience left us with some questions:

- How could this mishap occur?

  The researchers used a hypothesis that is incompatible with the assumptions underlying the input data set that comes with PREVENT. They viewed PREVENT as a *black box*, evidently not questioning results sufficiently, even when they seemed illogical.

- How serious is it?

  We think it is not very serious, because most readers will deem the conclusions unrealistic. However, the suggestion that these unrealistic estimates originate from PREVENT may have blemished PREVENT's reputation.

- Could it have been avoided?

  This question is much harder to answer. We did comment on a draft version of the final report and pointed out the problem, but the researchers chose to publish the results anyway. One might even get philosophical about it and formulate a corollary of Murphy's Law: *Whichever way a model can be abused, it will.* When you make expert knowledge available to non-experts, you should not expect them to become experts.

We learned from this experience that it is crucial to keep a close watch on serious applications of the model. In most cases this has proved unnecessary: most users apparently know what they are doing. And we are convinced that the benefits outweigh an occasional accident. But some accidents will happen. So the moral of this story is: when you distribute a model, be prepared for unexpected results.

Recommendations

Epidemiology has sometimes claimed to be a basic science for public health. Results from theoretical and empirical epidemiological work can, indeed, be used to provide information essential to public health decisions. To be of use for policy making, however, epidemiological data often need to be *interpreted.* Such applied epidemiology will often necessitate a simulation model. Global modelling for policy purposes with epidemiological data is possible and useful. Health policy making with such public health models can improve priority setting by providing more precise quantification of effect estimates, but it will also require precise target setting, and an investment in the collection of data which are essential to such an exercise.

This project was a first step on the road from aetiological and intervention research to the implementation of these results in health policy making. It shows that the health benefits of preventive interventions may differ from those expected from the traditional measures of effect. However, to make future results more realistic further research will be necessary, especially concerning the inclusion of possible changes in curative care in a more comprehensive public health model.

References

1. WHO (1985) Targets for Health for all. Targets in support of the European regional strategy for Health for All. World Health Organization, Regional Office for Europe, Copenhagen, pp 1-201
2. Gunning-Schepers LJ (1989) The health benefits of prevention, a simulation approach. Health Policy 12:1-256

3. Morgenstern H, Bursic ES (1982) A method for using epidemiologic data to estimate the potential impact of an intervention on the health status of a target population. Journal of Community Health 7:292-309
4. de Looijer FANM, Vrancken PHJ (1990) Efecten van fiscale harmonisatie in Europa op gezondheid en gezondheidszorg. Institute for Research on Public Spending, The Hague, pp 1-103
5. Parker DA, Harman MS (1978) The distribution of consumption model of prevention of alcohol problems. Journal of Studies on Alcohol 39:377-399

Modelling Latent Effects in any Association between Oral Contraceptives and Breast Cancer

K. McPherson

Introduction

The epidemiological results of investigations into a possible association between oral contraceptives (OC) and breast cancer appear quite conflicting. Several well-conducted cohort studies suggest rather strongly that long-term OC use is not associated with any change in breast cancer incidence, with the possible exception of one study. Most case control studies also indicate overall no particular grounds for concern, with some important exceptions. Vital statistics, in the form of mortality rates or registration rates, also are reassuring, but again with one or two non-trivial exceptions.

This paper reviews the epidemiological evidence to some extent, although its main purpose is to discuss the implication of particular kinds of biological mechanisms in interpreting the epidemiology. Epidemiological studies tend to be interpreted by assuming that a possible disease-causing mechanism has immediate effect. Thus it is assumed, often implicitly, that if OC use does have an effect on breast cancer, such an effect is essentially spontaneous. Therefore, any study which indicates no association is taken, perhaps mistakenly, to mean there is no causative effect, whereas a more precise interpretation might be that there is no effect which manifests itself immediately or in the short term. Clearly, such evidence does not exclude a delayed effect, unless much relevant exposure occurred a long time before the events recorded by the study.

For many chronic diseases, such as breast cancer, time delays between exposure to risk factors and diagnosis of disease may be as long as several decades. New and rapidly changing exposures, such as the use of OCs, may therefore be associated with great uncertainty in the interpretation of their epidemiological relationships. In the example discussed here, the implications are important, firstly because OC use is common and, secondly, because breast cancer is the most frequent female cancer among Western communities. Since a biological association is, a priori, highly plausible, the potential for a large ultimate attributable risk is extremely important.

Clearly, such uncertainties cannot finally be resolved until sufficient time has elapsed to enable definitive study of any delayed relationship. In the interim period, however, several investigations can throw important light on scientific and policy questions. These concern the modelling of plausible effects with a view to understanding their importance in contemporary epidemiology, so that current studies can be interpreted more completely. Until sufficient time has elapsed, the main problem will be a paucity of relevant data. It is therefore as well to understand the arguments against these hypotheses, and the precision of current studies. Finally, it is helpful to investigate the method of analysis that will reveal any delayed effects.

Above all, it is essential to know what kinds of effects are, or are not, consistent with the observed contemporary relationships. That is, to what extent are individual studies consistent with an important delayed effect, and to what extent are the many apparent inconsistencies due to a delayed effect.

Evidence about an Association between OCs and Breast Cancer

Many epidemiological studies have been made of the relationship between OC use and subsequent breast cancer risk. Most show no immediate association, and this evidence has been considered to be reassuring. Breast cancer is one of the commonest cancers among women in the developed world, and clearly has a hormonal aetiology. Hence any observed epidemiological association with OC use would be both plausible and extremely important.

Cohort studies, which were mostly begun in the 1960s, soon after OCs became available, have shown little cause for concern. They did not show long-term OC use to be associated with any change in breast cancer risk [1]. Only one cohort study [2] has reported an elevated risk of use of OCs, but only for breast cancer at a young age. A useful review of this association by Prentice and Thomas [3], using meta-analysis, shows a relative risk about unity for OC use and breast cancer risk. This appears to be true both among long-term OC users and among women using OCs ten to twenty years before diagnosis.

The overall summary of case control studies included in the review by Prentice and Thomas also suggested no extra risk associated with OC use for many years before diagnosis, but a relative risk of about 1.3 for prolonged use before first full-term pregnancy. Schlesselman [4] has also described an increasing risk with increasing duration of exposure before first full-term pregnancy, based on an average of all published studies.

Several case control studies have been published [5-9], which appear to show an association between OC use at a young age (described as early OC use) and breast cancer. But such studies are by no means unanimous, and several others [10-12] seem to show no association.

Women using OCs before first full-term pregnancy, or at a young age, clearly are an important subgroup in this context. However, it should be noted that it is a subgroup of the total exposed population and to some extent is data-derived. Many plausible subgroups could be investigated for this association, and this one has been emphasized partly for the reasons discussed.

The most recent results of the UK National Case-Control Study, among women under the age of 36, estimated a relative risk of up to 1.7 for eight years of total OC use. Being recent, it includes the most up-to-date information on the association for a high proportion of very young OC users. It is important to recognize that there is a necessary association between exposure to OCs at a young age and being currently young (see below).

The association of OCs and breast cancer could be of major public health significance if such risks, found among under-35 year olds, are not confined to this age. There have been large changes in the extent, timing, and type of OC use by different cohorts, so that any association of early OC use is difficult to study reliably. This is particularly so since OC use at different times in a woman's life may have quite different effects on breast cancer risk.

Some [13] have argued persuasively that the positive associations in the literature may be due to survey biases inherent in observational case control study methodology. It is difficult to exclude such an explanation from particular observational studies, and hence they remain plausible causes of some or all of the discrepancies. It is also possible, however, that the largest apparently negative study [11] has been incorrectly reported as being negative [14, 15].

The fact that recent worrying studies are all case control studies may reflect the fact that cohort studies, which were mostly started in the late sixties, concentrate on OC use at that time among women who were users then. Paradoxically, as we shall see, this may make them less relevant than contemporary case control studies.

The Possibility of Latent Effect

The notion that a latent effect could be important has received some attention [16, 17]. A latent interval could include an induction period, during which time a single cancer cell is evolving, and a pre-clinical period, the time between the first cancer cell and the diagnosis of cancer. If we examine epidemiological studies of breast cancer, several features emerge as being possibly relevant to an association with OCs. A relatively young age at menarche carries a higher risk [5], as does late age at first full-term pregnancy [18]. Breast cancer is very uncommon at ages younger than the mid-forties, and hence age at menarche or first child birth, if primary risk factors, must operate with a *latent* interval of thirty years or more in some cases.

Diethylstilboestrol (DES), a drug introduced in the 1940s and 50s to prevent miscarriage, has been shown to be associated with an increase in subsequent breast cancer incidence. One study [19], among 3 000 exposed women and 3 000 similar women who were not exposed to the drug, showed a relative risk of about 2 associated with exposure, after 40 years of follow-up. After 20 years there was no divergence in the cumulative breast cancer incidence curves between exposed and unexposed. Hence any epidemiological investigation undertaken among these women during the first 20 years after exposure would have shown an estimated relative risk of around unity.

It is therefore entirely plausible that OCs could be associated with a delayed effect on breast cancer incidence. Hence it remains plausible that contemporary epidemiology is yielding biased estimates of what may turn out to be the greatest relative risk. These may be termed *analytical* biases, as opposed to *survey* biases referred to by Skegg [13] since, if present, they arise from inadequate implied models of disease causation used in the analysis. Conventional statistical analysis implicitly assumes that exposure has an immediate effect on risk. If OCs affect early-stage carcinogenesis when used at a young age, or act as co-initiators by affecting mitotic activity [20], then any alteration in observed risk might not occur for 20 years or so after accumulated use. Anderson et al. [21] have demonstrated an increased rate of mitotic activity in the endothelial cells of the breast among young women taking OCs. This increase was confined to nulliparous women, hence a particular effect of OC use before first full-term pregnancy, for biological reasons, remains plausible.

Use Patterns of Oral Contraceptives

OCs have not been used in a consistent way since they were introduced in the early 1960s. At first, they were used largely by married women, mainly for family planning. This is because, at that time, it was difficult for unmarried women to be prescribed OCs. Patterns of use gradually changed during the early sixties, and later, during the *swinging sixties*, all sorts of cultural expectations and social behaviour changed dramatically. In the UK, the early seventies witnessed a sharp rise in the prevalence of OC use among teenagers; from around 15% of sexually active single women aged under 20 in 1970, to 50% by 1975, and nearly 80% by 1980 [22, 23]. During this period the dose has decreased, and the kinds of synthetic hormones used have changed.

The important point is that widespread use of OCs by women in their teens (described here as early use) is a recent phenomenon, and is more recent in some communities than in others. There is some evidence to suggest, for instance, that use of OCs by young women started in the USA more recently than in the UK [17, 24]. Very little can now be said about the effect of early OC use on breast cancer risk at age forty or over, simply because the women who have been exposed are only now reaching this age.

Simulation and Modelling

The Simulation Model

A computer programme was used to simulate individual exposure to OCs, and a subsequent diagnosis of breast cancer, in hypothetical cohorts of women *born* in each calendar year from 1930 to 1965. To estimate the prevalence of exposure to OCs, we analyzed the data from 2 246 controls included in case control studies of breast cancer, conducted in Oxford between 1968 and 1984. We also used data from the RCGP pilot study of contraception [25]. The controls were women who were matched within five years of age with breast cancer cases being treated in hospital; some were also matched by parity. The selection of controls is described in detail elsewhere [26]. We derived the distribution of these women who had been exposed to OCs before first full-term pregnancy by calendar year of birth (see Table 1).

Table 1. Early OC use (before full-time pregnancy) by birth cohort and duration (expressed as %)

OC use (years)	Year of birth 19-								
	≤29	30-34	35-39	40-44	45-49	50-54	55-59	60-64	65-69
0	99	97	94	86	59	43	5	4	17
<4	1	3	5	12	29	43	63	58	81
≥4	0	0	1	2	12	14	32	39	2
n	621	646	268	496	154	48	147	426	447

In the simulation, each woman was assigned randomly, according to those proportions, to one of three groups describing her exposure to OCs: never used, used for up to 4 years, or used for 4 or more years. Incorporated into the simulation were the England and Wales age-specific risks of breast cancer [14], so that each woman generated had the appropriate age-specific incidence applied to her. The incidence for a woman exposed to OCs was multiplied by a factor some time (the latent interval) after her exposure. We chose two hypothetical associations of early exposure with breast cancer incidence. The first assigned a relative risk of 1.4 to *up to 4 years' OC use* and 3.0 to *4 or more years' OC use*, and the second assigned double these risks, i.e. 2.8 and 6.0, respectively.

The latent interval determined the point after OC exposure at which the incidence of breast cancer was multiplied by this relative risk. Data on mean age at first OC use, by year of birth, were obtained by interpolation and extension of figures from OC use before first full-term pregnancy among controls in our studies. For any woman, age at first OC exposure was determined randomly from a Gaussian distribution with the appropriate mean, and a standard deviation of 4 years, subject to the constraints that this age was not less than 15 years, and that OCs had not been used before the year 1962. The time at which the latent interval began was arbitrarily taken as 3 years after the start of OC use for women with 0-4 years' exposure, and 5 years after the start for those with 4 or more years' exposure.

Five separate patterns of latency were considered. The first was no latent interval. The remaining four consisted of a variable latent interval with a Gaussian distribution and:

- mean 5 years, standard deviation 2 years
- mean 10 years, standard deviation 4 years
- mean 15 years, standard deviation 4 years
- mean 20 years, standard deviation 4 years.

A Gaussian distribution was chosen because latency could be the sum of several independent random time-delay processes, such as a sub-clinical period, a prolonged carcinogenic process, or the sum of the times between successive stages and the final stage in a multi-stage process. The stated standard deviations were chosen so that, at least for some average latencies, there was effectively a minimum latent period. The evidence already cited does suggest that no excess cancers in an exposed group need be observed for the first ten or fifteen years. An exponential and a lognormal distribution [27] with similar mean durations were also considered.

Cases of breast cancer were generated by this micro simulation. For each case thus generated, a random control without breast cancer was selected, of the same age and fully comparable with respect to all other risk factors except OC use. These matched pairs were then used for the analysis of simulated matched case control studies, conducted at particular times up to the end of this century and among women of particular ages.

Results

This model can thus provide insights into how latency can confuse the interpretation of epidemiology. The extent of the effect is surprising, and might even be considered alarming, in the absence of hard evidence. However, while some studies show no evidence of a delayed effect, others do [9, 28]. The apparent conflict between studies could be due to differences in the time at which early OC use became common among young women. If, for example, such use is more recent in one country than in another, then obviously, if there is a latent effect, the estimated relative risks may be correspondingly different.

Straightforward statistical arguments indicate that contemporary studies of this association will lack precision if the delay period is around 20 years, because it is rare to find relevant exposure which occurred sufficiently long ago. In one recent study [28], only 1.4% of 351 controls aged less than 45 had used OCs prior to first full-term pregnancy more than 20 years before the diagnosis of their age-matched case. This represented only five women, none of whom, moreover, had accumulated prolonged use by this time. Thus such apparent inconsistency is consistent with a latent effect.

In general, if there were an effect of the kind described above, then the observed relative risk associated with a given exposure would be expected, firstly, to increase with increasing age at diagnosis and, secondly, to increase as recent exposure was omitted. Both of these characteristics are true of two recent studies. For example, in the most recent National study, the estimated relative risk increased with age, from 1.5 at age less than 30 to 2.0 at age 34-35. Moreover, as recent OC use is excluded as an exposure variable, so the estimated relative risk increases.

If, for instance, one postulates that long-term use of OCs before first full-term pregnancy ultimately increases the risk of breast cancer threefold, but that the time between this effect and diagnosis is 15 years, with a standard deviation of 4 years, then studies which include women of different age-groups, based on OC use patterns shown in Table 1, should yield estimates of relative risk as shown in Table 2.

The recent estimate of a relative risk of 1.3 for four years of OC use among women under the age of 35 is wholly consistent with an ultimate risk of three and a delay of only 15 years, on average, between accumulated exposure and diagnosis. This was almost exactly the risk observed in the UK National study from 1982 to 1985.

Table 2. Estimated relative risk of ≥ 4 years' early exposure among women of different ages if the latent interval is Gaussian with mean and standard deviations as shown, and if the ultimate relative risk is three

Latent period (years) Mean	sd	Age 25-29	30-34	35-39	40-44
None		3.0	3.0	3.0	3.0
5	2	1.8	2.2	3.0	3.0
10	4	1.0	1.9	2.3	2.7
15	4	1.0	1.3	1.8	2.3
20	4	1.0	1.0	1.3	1.4

Similarly, if the use patterns by birth cohort shown in Table 1 are a true reflection of actual use in the UK, then the estimated relative risk observed in case control studies, including only women of such an age as to have been exposed while young, would progress as in Figure 1 if the average latent interval is 15 years. The confidence limits in Figure 1 reflect the increasing age of breast cancer cases and controls who may have been exposed while young, as time progresses.

Thus increasing power will become available to test these hypotheses. A full tabulation of the point estimates under the various assumptions is shown in Table 3.

If this model is at all realistic, then cancer incidence will only change gradually as the cohort of women who have used OCs for prolonged periods while young reach an age where breast cancer becomes relatively common. Simulations again indicate the extent of this effect, using exactly the same assumptions as before. Because patterns of early OC use change with time, the predicted changes among particular age-groups might be as shown in Table 4. It can be seen that only small changes in incidence would be expected, even if the relative risk were ultimately as high as three.

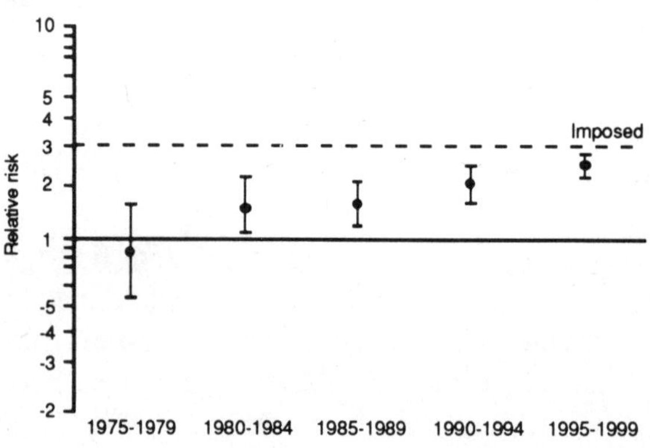

Fig. 1. *Unbiased* estimates of relative risk of ≥ 4 years of early OC use relative to calendar time, if an effect is delayed by an average of 15 years with a standard deviation of 4 years

This is an unsatisfactory state of affairs, because no detectable change in the incidence by 1985 might be expected, even if there is an important as-

Table 3. Estimated relative risk of ≥4 years of OC use with calendar time, including only women who have been, or will be, exposed, if the true relative risk is three

Latent period (years)		Calendar period				
Mean	sd	1975-1979	1980-1984	1985-1989	1990-1994	1995-1999
None		3.0	3.0	3.0	3.0	3.0
5	2	2.4	2.6	2.7	3.0	3.0
10	4	1.6	1.4	2.1	2.8	3.0
15	4	1.2	1.6	1.8	2.1	2.6
20	4	1.0	1.0	1.1	1.6	2.0

sociation. Incidence figures which have been published for 1985 are not inconsistent with Table 4. There are some increases among young women, which are not consistent or worrying in themselves.

Fortunately, recent work from New Zealand [29] contradicts these pessimistic arguments but does not refute them, because the power against plausible risks remains very low. The massive CASH study from the USA is often cited as strong evidence against such an effect, based on the assumption that it showed no effect of early OC use [15]. It is no longer clear that it does [14], although clarification is still awaited. Moreover, the evidence does suggest that early OC use started about five years later in the USA, and as the study was done in the early 1980s, an estimated relative risk of unity must

Table 4. Percentage increase in incidence of breast cancer among women of different ages attributable to early OC use, if the ultimate relative risk associated with such use is three, with an average delay of 15 years

	Age			
Year	35-39	40-44	45-49	50-54
1981	0	0	0	0
1982	1	1	0	0
1983	2	1	0	0
1984	5	2	0	0
1985	7	4	1	0
1986	10	5	2	0
1987	13	6	3	1
1988	17	9	5	1
1989	21	12	7	2
1990	25	16	10	3
1995	41	36	31	14
2000	52	68	53	42

be interpreted like an estimated relative risk of unity in 1975 in the UK. Both are wholly consistent with an ultimate relative risk of three, combined with a latent period of 15 years.

The analytical methods for investigating a latent effect involve manipulation of the definition of exposure. Normally, in studies of OC use and chronic disease, a category of exposure is defined such as *four or more years of use before first full-term pregnancy*. Thus subjects either do or do not fall into this category; the relative risks are calculated from the numbers of cases and control, in each exposure category. As already indicated, such analyses assume there is an immediate effect.

If one wishes to investigate a latent effect, then clearly the exposure variable must take on another dimension of definition which reflects the temporal relationship between exposure and disease, for example *four or more years of use more than ten years before diagnosis*. In matched case control studies, such a definition can be accommodated by taking the diagnosis date for the case, and the date when the control was the same age as the matched case at time of diagnosis. When investigating a latent effect, and when one has little prior information about the length of the latent interval, it is better progressively to extend the period between exposure and diagnosis. Thus OC use within two years of diagnosis is first excluded, then within four years, and so on. On each occasion the categories of duration will change, as parts of the total duration of OC use are excluded.

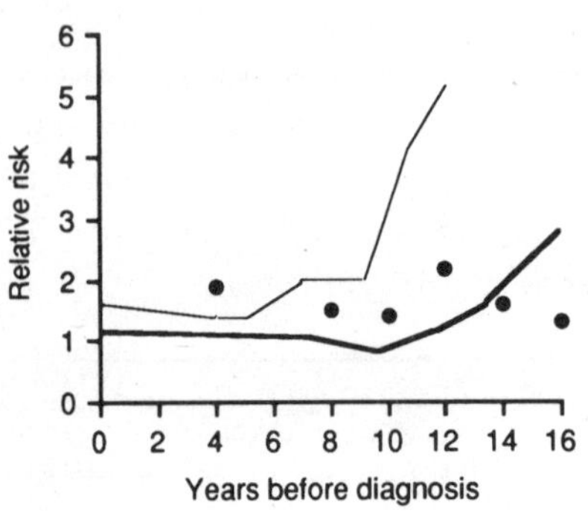

Fig. 2. Estimated relative risk of ≥ 4 years of early OC use when excluding accumulated use prior to diagnosis for cases, and the equivalent date for controls. The black line represents simulations for a hypothetical study conducted in 1980-1984 with a true relative risk of 3.0 and an average delay of 15 years, and the dotted line represents a relative risk of 6. The black dots represent the actual analysis of McPherson et al., 1987 [6] for OC use before first pregnancy. Since the data are sparse, however, the confidence limits on every dot include the simulation lines.

In this way, a latent effect would manifest itself by an increasing estimate of relative risk as recent use was progressively excluded. Using the simulation model such an effect can be seen in Figure 2. Each period on the abscissa represents increasing exclusion. To investigate such an effect in real life is straightforward in principle, but the data are as yet extremely sparse for the reasons discussed.

References

1. Mann RD (ed) (1990) Oral Contraceptions and Breast Cancer. Parthenon, Carnforth Lancs
2. Royal College of General Practitioners (1988) Breast cancer and the pill - A further report from the Royal College of General Practitioners study. Brit J Cancer 58:675-680
3. Prentice RL, Thomas DB (1987) On the epidemiology of oral contraceptives and disease. Advances in Cancer Research 49:285-401
4. Schesselman JJ (1989) Oral contraceptives in relation to cancer of the breast and reproductive tract. An epidemiological review. Contraception 40:1
5. Pike MC, Krailo MD, Henderson BE, Cosagrande JT, Hoel DG (1983) Hormonal risk factors for breast cancer. Nature 303:767-770
6. McPherson K, Vessey MP, Neil A, Doll R, Jones L, Roberts M (1987) Early oral contraceptive use and breast cancer: Results of another case-control study. Brit J Cancer 56:653-660
7. Meirik O, Lund E, Adami HO, Bergstrim R, Christofferson T, Bergsjo P (1986) Oral contraceptive use and breast cancer in young women. Lancet ii:650-655
8. Miller DR, Rosenberg L, Kaufman DW, Stolley PD, Warshauer ME, Shapiro S (1989) Breast cancer before age 45 and oral contraceptive use: New findings. Amer J Epidemiol 129:269-280
9. UK National Case-Control Study Group (1989) Oral contraceptive use and breast cancer in young women. Lancet:973-982
10. Paul C, Skegg DCG, Spears CFS, Kalder JM (1986) Oral contraceptives and breast cancer: A National study. Brit Med J 293:723-728
11. Stadel BV, Robin GL, Webster L, Sclesselman JJ, Wing PA (1985) Oral contraceptives and breast cancer in young women. Lancet ii:970-974
12. Miller DR, Rosenberg L, Kaufman DW, Schottenfeld D, Stolley PD, Shapiro S (1986) Breast cancer risk in relation to early oral contraceptive use. J Obst Gynaecol:863-868
13. Skegg DCG (1988) Potential for bias in case-control studies of oral contraceptives and breast cancer. Amer J Epidemiol 127:205-211
14. Peto J (1989) Is the CASH study really negative? Lancet i (11 March 1989):552
15. Stadel B, Schlesselman JJ, Murray PA (1989) Oral contraceptives and breast cancer. Lancet (3 June 1989):1257-1258
16. McPherson, K Coope PA, Vessey MP (1986) Early oral contraceptive use and breast cancer - theoretical effects of latency. Brit J Epidemiol and Comm Health 40:289-294
17. McPherson K (1988) Latent effect of oral contraceptives on breast cancer. JAMA 260:1240-1241
18. McMahan B, Cole P, Brown J (1973) Etiology of human breast cancer. A review. J Nat Cancer Inst 50:21-32
19. Greenberg ER, Barnes AB, Ressequie L, Barrat JA, Burndide S, Lanza LL, Neff RR, Stevens M, Young RH, Colton T (1984) Breast cancer in mothers given diethylstibestrol in pregnancy. New Eng J Med 311:1393-1397

20. Buehring GC (1988) Oral contraceptives and breast cancer: what has 20 years of research shown? Biomed and Pharmac 42:525-530
21. Anderson TJ, Battersby S, King RJB, McPherson K (1989) Breast epithelial responses and steroid receptors during oral contraceptive use. Hum Pathol 12:1137-1143
22. Dunnell K (1976) Family Formation. OPCS, HMSO, London
23. Bone M, (1978) The family planning services: changes and effects. OPCS, HMSO, London
24. Bachrach CA (1984) Contraceptive practice among young American women, 1973-1982. Family Planning Perspectives 16 (6):253-259
25. Kay C (1986) Steroidal contraceptive pilot study report. Royal College of General Practitioners, London
26. Vessey MP, Doll R, Sutton PM (1972) Oral contraceptives and breast neoplasia: A retrospective study. Br Med J 3:719-724
27. Armenian HK, Lilienfeld AM (1983) Incubation periods of disease. Epidemiol Rev 5:1-15
28. McPherson K (1990) Summary and update of the Oxford-based studies. In: Mann RD (ed) Oral contraceptives and breast cancer. Parthenon, Carnforth, pp 55-66
29. Paul C, Skegg DCG (1990) Oral contraceptives and breast cancer in New Zealand. In: Man RD (ed) Oral contraceptives and breast cancer. Parthenon, Carnforth, pp 85-94

Diabetes Population Projections

F. Hauser and M. Andel

Introduction

Diabetes mellitus is rarely the immediate cause of death, but is an important underlying factor leading to the main cause of death. The late clinical complications of diabetes cause a substantial deterioration in the quality of life, and the disease represents an important risk factor for a number of serious illness, such as atherosclerosis, renal failure, and hepatitis B.

The number of diabetics is continuously growing throughout the world, but the reasons for this are not yet entirely clear. However, those concerned with health care planning and financing would like to have reasonably reliable forecasts in order to ensure that the necessary resources are available. Diabetics need, above all, antidiabetic drugs, diagnostic instruments and materials, therapeutic instruments, certain high-technology facilities, and well-trained medical personnel.

Future health care needs can be estimated in various ways. Any sophisticated approach must take into account the health status of the population, which for diabetes can be expressed in terms of the incidence and prevalence of the disease and the mortality of diabetics. Forecasts of diabetes prevalence can then serve as a basis for estimating needed resources.

The most often used types of health projections have been surveyed by Lopez and Hakama [1]. Apart from subjective methods (e.g. the Delphi method), and methods based on the processing of a single variable (time-series extrapolation), most health projections are concerned with either incidence or mortality. The models used in such projections incorporate the effects of other variables which are thought to represent risk factors for the disease in question.

Several authors have studied the combined effect of incidence and mortality trends on changes in prevalence. Simple models of this type were developed at the International Institute for Applied Systems Analysis (IIASA), for studying the epidemiology of lung cancer, chronic obstructive lung disease, and ischaemic heart disease [2, 3, 4]. An example of a rather complex model is the work of Parkin on cervical cancer [5]. In diabetology this approach was used by Herman et al. [6], based on a very rough age structure, and by us [7].

The Model

The evolution of the diabetic population is described by means of a medico-demographic simulation model. Medical aspects of the population structure were added to the type of population projection commonly used in demography. The population is classified, not only by sex and age, but also by health status.

The population projection is calculated by the programme MULTISPOM [8]. This represents a compartmental model described by difference equations. Using time steps of one year, it calculates the yearly evolution of the age-sex structure of a population, divided into several categories of health status. These categories have to be defined so that each is directly related to at least one other category, and so that each member of the study population can be assigned to just one category at any given moment. Individuals can move from one health status category to another, the transition rates being determined by coefficients which, in general, are dependent on external factors.

Untreated diabetes mellitus is diagnosed by chronic elevation of the concentration of glucose in the blood (hyperglycaemia) [9]. In reality, however, diabetes is the symptom of several distinct diseases due to several causes. Although a fully satisfactory classification has not yet been created, the one adopted by the WHO Expert Committee on Diabetes Mellitus is generally accepted. This distinguishes two main types of diabetes mellitus: insulin-dependent (Type 1) and non-insulin-dependent (Type 2) [9]. Despite some diagnostic problems, each type has a different aetio-pathogenesis, and consequently a different incidence, prevalence, and mortality. Differences also exist in risk factors, genetics, possibilities of prevention, and therapy.

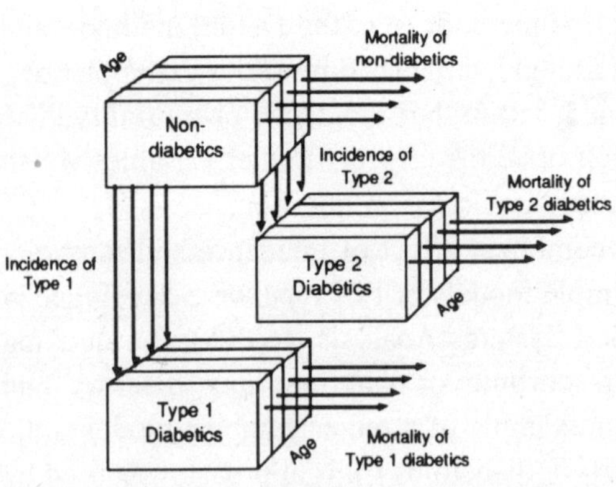

Fig. 1. A medico-demographic model of diabetes

The model takes these differences into account, and distinguishes three health status categories (Fig. 1): Type 1 diabetics, Type 2 diabetics, and non-diabetics. In the first year of the projection, the complete population composition by age, sex, and health status category has to be specified. For this purpose, the number of people in the general population, and the prevalence of the two types of diabetes must be known. In calculating the population structure for the following year, the model takes into account age-specific fertilities in each health status category, the sex ratio of newborn babies, perinatal mortality, and the probability of being born in a particular health category. Transitions between health categories are determined by age- and sex-specific incidence and mortality rates.

Prevalence and Incidence of Diabetes

The epidemiology of Type 1 diabetes has been studied in many European countries. Most studies of its prevalence and incidence cover the age range from birth to 14 or 19 years, and few extend to 29 years. Surveys of some recent studies can be found [10, 11]. Significant geographical differences have been found in Europe, with a higher incidence and prevalence in the north than in the south. Increasingly detailed data are becoming available as computer registries are established. It is apparent that registries of Type 1 patients are highly suitable for epidemiological studies, because almost all cases can be identified by routine methods.

Very few studies, in Europe or elsewhere, have been made of Type 2 diabetes. The main reason is the difficulty of identifying cases in the population according to WHO criteria [12]. Incidence was studied in the UK by Barker et al. [13] and in Sweden by Ostman et al. [14]. In some countries prevalence was estimated, but in fairly small regions. In the former German Democratic Republic (GDR) and in Czechoslovakia, Type 2 diabetics have been registered and dispensed treatment, and a system of reporting has provided prevalence data, for many years. A more elaborate system in the former GDR provided age-specific prevalence and incidence rates of the two diabetes types [15].

Incidence might depend on certain risk factors, but most risk factors for diabetes are known only on a qualitative level. When quantitative information, confirmed by several studies, becomes available, the model will have to be made more detailed to include it. This is the case for the HLA-DR3 and/or HLA-DR4 alleles of the major histocompability complex in Europeans, an established risk factor for Type 1 diabetes, or for obesity, an established risk factor for Type 2 diabetes. As the model becomes more complex, however, other data become necessary which are less readily available.

Mortality of Diabetics

Of the three epidemiological variables - prevalence, incidence, and mortality - mortality is the most troublesome. It is generally accepted that the mortality of diabetics exceeds the mortality in the general population, but reliable quantitative data are difficult to obtain.

Treatment of children with Type 1 diabetes has substantially improved since the introduction of insulin in 1922. Nevertheless, mortality remains significantly higher than in non-diabetics [16]. Before the introduction of insulin the mortality was 386 per 1 000, and the average life expectancy after diagnosis was only 1 or 2 years. After insulin therapy came into use, the mortality dropped to 61 per 1 000 within four years [17]. The mortality has been decreasing ever since, but is still about seven times higher than that of non-diabetic children [18]. Similar excess mortality has been found up to middle age [19, 20], and a marked increase was observed after the age of 35.

Continuous improvement in the mortality complicates the evaluation of long-term prospective follow-up studies, which would otherwise be expected to provide the best results. One problem with the use of long-term studies or those performed long ago [21, 22] is classification. In studies performed before the WHO classification was adopted, age at diagnosis was the only criterion for determining diabetes type [23].

Most studies of mortality of Type 2 diabetics classify patients according to age at diagnosis. A rare exception is the Finnish prospective study by Reunanen [24]. A further problem with Type 2 diabetes is that some cases are unaware of their disorder. A survey of all-cause mortality studies published before 1986 was made by Panzram [23].

From the viewpoint of the model shown in Figure 1, most studies of diabetes mortality have certain drawbacks. The most serious is that the presented mortalities are not age-specific. Age dependence is sometimes considered, but data are presented in an inconvenient form such as cumulative mortality or survivorship. Finally, many articles provide data only on cause-specific mortalities, most often on coronary heart disease or cerebrovascular disease. Mortality data for the model thus remain a big challenge.

Until now, there has been little information relating potential risk factors to subsequent mortality of diabetics. The few results available suggest that mortality risk factors are not significantly different in diabetic and non-diabetic populations [25].

Conclusions

Attempts to make projections for the diabetic population have two aspects. One is to study the kinetics of this population and unravel the nature of its growth. The other is to forecast, as reliably as possible, future population size as a basis for the objective assessment of health care needs.

The approach to projection which we adopted is based on disease prevalence calculated from age- and sex-specific incidence and mortality rates. This approach implies certain special requirements for epidemiological data, and requires some knowledge of aetiology. Expert knowledge and assumptions have to be used to complement or substitute for weak or absent epidemiological data.

By specifying new data requirements, the modelling process contributes to the development of a health care information system, and helps in the planning of further epidemiological studies. The health care information system itself is rapidly improving, owing to developments in computers and computer networks, with ever-increasing access to growing amounts of disaggregated data. These conditions favour the construction of more detailed epidemiological models, which more closely represent reality.

In the case of diabetes, attempts should be made to study regional differences in incidence and try to explain them. A much deeper knowledge is needed about risk factors related to the incidence of diabetes and the mortality of diabetics. Of major importance is the identification of those factors which could be influenced by primary prevention programmes.

The rising cost of drugs is causing increasing concern among those who are responsible for health care financing and planning. Drug consumption depends on a number of factors, the most important of which is the population's health status. Projections of the diabetic population provide the most direct way of estimating the need for diabetic care. This has led to practical applications of the model. The model has been quantified for the Czech Republic, and the diabetic population projection has been used for estimating the future needs of insulin [26] and oral hypoglycaemic drugs [27].

References

1. Lopez AD, Hakama M (1986) Approaches to projections of health status. In: Health projections in Europe: methods and applications. WHO Regional Office for Europe, Copenhagen, pp 9-24
2. Rusnak M, Yashin A, Merinska I (1986) Smoking and lung cancer prevalence: Slovakian case study. IIASA, Laxenburg, pp 11-23
3. Rusnak M, Yashin A, Kristufek P (1985) The future of lung diseases: COPD model for Slovakia. IIASA, Laxenburg, pp 10-21
4. Koonce JF, Yashin AI, Walters CJ, Rusnak M (1984) Modelling of public health: call for interdisciplinary actions. IIASA, Laxenburg, pp 22-38
5. Parkin D (1985) A computer simulation model for the practical planning of cervical cancer screening programmes. Brit J Cancer 51:551-568

6. Herman WL, Sinnock P, Brenner E, Brimberry JL, Langford D, Nakashima A, Sepe SJ, Teutsch SM, Mazze RS (1984) An epidemiological model for diabetes mellitus: incidence prevalence and mortality. Diabetes Care 7:367-371
7. Hauser F, Andel M (1988) Projection of the prevalence of type 1 and type 2 diabetes. In: Carson ER, Kneppo P, Krekule I (eds) Advances in Biomedical Measurement. Plenum, New York, pp 407-413
8. Mader R (1986) A model for prognosing population age structure evolution in several health state phases. Cs zdravotnictv 34:218-224
9. WHO (1985) Diabetes Mellitus. WHO Technical Report Series No 727, Geneva, pp 9-20
10. Zimmet P, King H (1985) The epidemiology of diabetes mellitus: recent developments. In: Alberti KGMM, Krall LP (eds) The Diabetes Annual-1. Elsevier, Amsterdam, pp 1-15
11. Rewers M, LaPorte RE, King H, Tuomilehto J (1989) Trends in the prevalence and incidence of diabetes: Insulin-dependent diabetes mellitus in childhood. Wld Hlth Statist Quart 41:179-189
12. King H, Zimmet P (1988) Trends in the prevalence and incidence of diabetes: Non-insulin-dependent diabetes mellitus. Wld Hlth Statist Quart 41:190-196
13. Barker DJP, Gardner MJ, Power C (1982) Incidence of diabetes amongst people aged 18-50 years in nine British towns: a collaborative study. Diabetologia 22:421-425
14. Ostman J, Arnquist H, Blohme G, Lithner F, Littorin B, Nyström L, Sandström A, Schersten B, Wall S, Wibell L (1986) Epidemiology of diabetes mellitus in Sweden. Results of the first year of a prospective study in the population age-group 15-34 years. Acta Med Scand 220:437-445
15. (1986) Das Gesundheitswesen der DDR. Institut für Sozialhygiene und Organisation des Gesundheitsschutzes, Berlin, pp 87-93
16. Scibilia J, Finegold D, Dorman J, Becker D, Drash A (1986) Why do children with diabetes die? Acta endocrinologica 113 (Suppl 279):326-333
17. Marks HH (1965) Longevity and mortality of diabetics. Amer J Publ Hlth 55:416-423
18. Dorman JS, Laporte RE, Kuller LH, Cruickshanks KJ, Orchard TJ, Wagener DK, Becker DJ, Cavender DE, Drash AL (1984) The Pittsburgh insulin-dependent diabetes mellitus (IDDM) morbidity and mortality study: Mortality results. Diabetes 33:271-276
19. Connell FA (1985) Epidemiologic approaches to the identification of problems in diabetes care. Diabetes Care 8 (Suppl 1):82-86
20. Deckert T, Poulsen JE, Larsen M (1978) Prognosis of diabetics with diabetes onset before the age of thirty-one: I. Survival, causes of death and complications. Diabetologia 14:363-370
21. Kessler II (1971) Mortality experience of diabetic patients: A 26-year follow-up study. Amer J Med 51:715-724
22. Palumbo PJ (1976) Diabetes mellitus: Incidence, prevalence, survivorship, and causes of death in Rochester, Minnesota, 1945-1970. Diabetes 25:566-573
23. Panzram G (1987) Mortality and survival in Type 2 (non-insulin-dependent) diabetes mellitus. Diabetologia 30:123-131

24. Reunanen A (1983) Mortality in Type 2 diabetes. Ann Clin Res 15 (Suppl 37):26-28

25. Jarrett RJ, Shipley MJ (1985) Mortality and associated risk factors in diabetics. Acta Endocrinologica 110 (Suppl 272):21-26

26. Hauser F, Andel M (1988) Diabetic population projection and its use for estimating insulin need. In: Duru G, Engelbrecht R, Flagle CD, van Eimeren W (eds) System Science in Health Care. Masson 3, Paris, pp 35-38

27. Hauser F, Andel M, Honzakova L, Stika L (1990) Prognosis of the need of oral antidiabetics in the Czech Republic. Cas lek ces 129:129-34

Mortality and Morbidity Projections: Lung Cancer

M. Rusnak, S. Scherbov and B. Cider

Introduction

The health status of a population is a matter of growing interest to all those concerned with medical services. Many factors will affect the demand for health services up to the year 2000. A deep understanding of the relationships between factors which contribute to increases in morbidity is essential in order to influence the overall health of the population effectively. The health situation in rich countries is determined by a rising prevalence of noncommunicable diseases, despite a decline in mortality for some, e.g. cardiovascular diseases. Similar features are now emerging in other countries concerning the epidemiology of noncommunicable diseases, even in regions where communicable diseases are still the most important ones. Epidemiology, hand in hand with clinical medicine, is providing a growing amount of new information. The efforts and resources spent on collecting data are enormous. Multi-centre controlled intervention trials last for several years and require substantial investments in manpower, technology, and money. However, the benefits derived for clinical and health care management procedures do not keep pace with the growth of new information. Methods for applying the evidence which is collected for health care management are still being developed, and only a few of them are in daily routine use.

As a result of intensive epidemiological research carried out during the last 20 years, it is now generally accepted that lung cancer is a disease of modern civilization, and is largely preventable. In the first decade of this century, lung cancer was an uncommon tumour. This is in sharp contrast with facts from the last ten years. In 1977, the World Health Organization reported that, in many countries, death rates from cancers other than lung cancer were either stationary or declining in both males and females. In 1979, the American Cancer Society reported that the overall incidence of cancer had decreased slightly over the past 25 years, but that there was an increased death rate in men, mainly the result of lung cancer.

The aetiological factors in lung cancer are divided into personal air pollutants (smoking) and non-personal ones (which include atmospheric contaminants and industrial exposure). Tobacco smoking is considered to be the most potent aetiological factor in the development of bronchogenic carcinoma. The suggestion that smoking, and cigarette smoking in particular, may be important in the incidence of lung cancer has been made by many authors, even though controlled and large-scale clinical studies are lacking. The incidence of lung neoplasms correlates directly with population density, urbanization, industrialization, and tobacco smoking.

All the facts mentioned above suggest that we are facing a real epidemic of lung cancer. Obviously we are interested in the future evolution of this process. The most important questions are: how effective could preventive campaigns be, assuming different approaches? Where should preventive efforts be concentrated: on the younger or the older part of a population, on men or women, on smokers or non-smokers? A mathematical description of processes taking place in the affected population could help in answering such questions, and in forecasting future developments in epidemiology of the disease.

We have used the effects of smoking on lung cancer development to illustrate two different methods of projecting the future development of mortality and morbidity in a country. The first method is based on a multi-state population model, and the second on a simple matrix model. Both models provide a user-friendly man-machine interface, based on menus and windows.

Multi - State Approach

The IIASA Population Program has studied the possible changes in morbidity and mortality associated with a reduction in the prevalence of smoking. The first model for this purpose was developed at IIASA in 1986 [1]. Since then greater experience with the model has been acquired, new data have been collected, and the idea of a new model arose. The idea of using a multi-state approach, originally developed for demographic purposes, arose from discussions with demographers at the IIASA. Multi-state population models have recently become popular in studies of many aspects of demographic transitions, such as migration, marriage, and changes in health status, social status, and occupation. Previous experience with demographic applications of the DIALOG model [2], with its user-friendly man-machine interface, supported the idea of applying it to the study of lung cancer mortality and morbidity.

The effect of smoking on morbidity, mortality, and life expectancy was studied on data from Slovakia. The results of expected changes in the smoking population were forecast. With these forecasts, it is possible to predict the possible long-term effects of interventions, plan anti-smoking campaigns, and evaluate smoking control programmes.

DIALOG System

The DIALOG software system for multi-regional, multi-state population projections has resulted from methodological research being done at the International Institute for Applied System Analysis (IIASA), in collaboration with the All-Union Research Institute of Systems Studies, in Moscow [2]. The model is based on a mathematical description of multi-state population dynamics. It provides opportunities to prepare alternative scenarios, vary the parameters of the model during the modelling procedure, and obtain intermediate results. The system uses a simple, menu-based command language. It allows the user to control the modelling procedure, displays the results in a variety of forms, and permits flexible scenario setting.

The DIALOG system is modular in design. This allows flexibility in updating the system, and in changing old modules or adding new ones to the system to solve different tasks. The demographic model itself is represented as a separate unit. The control module generates the main table of model variables, switches control between other modules, and checks the memory distribution. All modules are interconnected through the control module.

During model initialization, the file with the initial data is read. The initialization unit calls the demographic model, and all variables of the model are calculated for the initial year. This allows the user to analyze demographic indicators for the first year, immediately after initialization. The scenario setting module provides for control of certain variables in the form of time series. In DIALOG, the control variables (or scenario variables) are the exogenous parameters of the demographic model used by the model at each simulation step. The set of control variables which is defined for a given time interval is called a scenario. Scenario setting can be performed in the interactive mode, or by calling a previously stored file. There is also an option to store scenarios, which were set in the interactive mode, in a file for future use. To the extent that scenario variables depend on a particular model, a scenario is set using variable names. There is also an opportunity to set scenarios for the main demographic indicators, such as life expectancy, total fertility rate, etc., without using special names for variables. After the user has defined all exogenous variables, their values are entered in a special table. At each step during simulation, all scenario variables are assigned values in accordance with their definition prior to calling the demographic model. Each new initialization of the model cancels the previously set scenario.

The simulation module provides the following functions at each step of simulation: for the current time, it assigns values for scenario variables, calls the demographic model, and controls simulation. A simulation step coincides with length of age cohort, while the simulation interval may consist of one or more simulation steps. Simulation can be performed for several time intervals. After completing the simulation of one time interval, the user may define the final time for the next time interval.

The data representation module presents data either at each simulation step (by writing data in the results file), or for the current time at the end of a simulation interval (output is to the terminal's screen). Information is presented in the form of tables and graphs. The DIALOG system was designed for IBM personal computers or compatibles.

The data used in the simulation of lung cancer were from the Slovak Socialist Republic of Czechoslovakia (Slovakia). Data from Slovakia were used because reliable data on smoking were available from a recent population survey, and data on lung cancer incidence and mortality were also available. The principal source of population data used was the official demographic statistical yearbook for Czechoslovakia, 1983. The data on smoking were from a survey on smoking in Slovakia done by Katriak et al. [3]. The coefficients for the transition from smoker to quitter were estimated from the results of the Hammond study of ex-smokers [4]. Information on the risk of lung cancer was lacking for Slovakia, so we used the results of a case-control interview study of lung cancer carried out in five European countries [5]. The data on lung cancer risk for non-smokers were taken from Enstrom [6].

Table1. Types of DIALOG output

Tables	Graphics
Age-specific rates	Population histogram
Gross rates	Age-specific fertility
Expectancies	Age-specific mortality
Birth, deaths	Pie chart by state
Transition flows	Population pyramid
Population by special age	
Category	
Summary table	
Population distribution	
% population distribution	

Results

The model was run first for basic projection. Projection from 1983 to 2003 was done without any changes to parameters. We tried to see how the lung cancer situation would appear if no changes were introduced during the period covered by the simulation. The results of the simulation can be displayed in tabular or graphical form. Table 1 gives a summary of possible outputs.

The change in gross mortality rates over time for all four states is summarized in Table 2.

Life expectancies at birth for people remaining in each of the four states are displayed in Table 3. When no scenario was introduced, there were no changes in life expectancies over the years of simulation. The only noticeable changes were in total life expectancy; this was due to a change in the sex ratio.

Table 4 shows the proportions of people in four states and in the years 1983 and 2013. The tendency for males to quit smoking, in contrast to females who keep on smoking, is reflected in the projected data. A similar feature has been observed in many other European countries.

Table 2. Gross mortality rates for all states in the initial year, and projection to year 2013

State	Year 1983	2013
Nonsmokers	2.920	2.906
Smokers	4.461	4.176
Quitters	3.158	3.072
Lung cancer	21.866	21.627

Table 3. Life expectancies at birth (years) for people in different states

State	Male	Female	Total
Nonsmokers	38.416	45.348	42.448
Smokers	14.565	10.455	12.635
Quitters	10.344	14.727	11.559
Lung cancer	0.077	0.077	0.060
Total	63.403	70.557	66.702

Conclusions

The main lesson to be drawn from the results presented above is that it is rational to use a model to describe the epidemiological characteristics of chronic diseases, and lung cancer in particular. The major problem encountered is non-availability of data. A typical situation is that not all the data required by the model are at hand. We had to use data from other countries, as well as expert estimates. The results of the Seven Countries Study [7] showed that, for cardiovascular diseases, predictions from one region are reasonably accurate for another region if similar conditions apply in both regions. Although the diversity of initial data resources has led to some discrepancies in projections, the results seem plausible as indicators of general trends in a population. The possibility of introducing a different scenario may be of value to the researcher who wishes to study the effects of assumed changes or interventions, although it was not attempted in this paper.

Table 4. Observed and projected proportions (%) of nonsmokers, smokers, quitters, and lung cancer cases in three age-groups, by sex

		Year					
		1983			2013		
State	Sex	0-14	15-64	≥65	0-14	15-64	≥65
Nonsmokers	M	51.0	43.0	6.0	40.7	54.6	4.7
	F	31.6	56.4	12.0	31.8	55.6	12.6
	T	39.1	51.2	9.7	35.7	55.2	9.2
Smokers	M	3.3	90.6	6.1	1.6	92.4	6.0
	F	2.5	93.9	3.6	3.1	91.4	5.5
	T	3.0	91.6	5.4	2.2	92.0	5.8
Quitters	M	0.8	77.8	21.4	0.1	78.1	21.8
	F	1.2	84.9	13.9	0.1	84.0	15.8
	T	0.9	80.5	18.6	0.1	81.0	18.8
Lung cancer	M	0.1	35.2	64.7	0.0	33.0	67.0
	F	0.0	22.1	77.9	0.0	19.0	81.0
	T	0.0	34.0	65.9	0.0	30.6	69.4

LCA Model

With the aim of forecasting lung cancer morbidity based on risk factors, we developed a dedicated model of lung cancer incidence, mortality, and prevalence forecasts, depending on the smoking habits of a population. The proposed model is based on the following assumptions:

- Smoking of cigarettes is generally recognized to be the principal cause of lung cancer. We treat this factor as the only one which causes lung cancer. This assumption has led us to ignore other possible aetiological factors, such as air pollution and alcohol abuse, which have not yet been definitely proved, but it allows us to emphasize the important role of anti-smoking campaigns in reducing the disease.

- Many different smoking habits exist: cigarettes or other types of smoking; low, medium, or high-tar cigarettes; the depth of inhalation, etc. This model takes no account of such differences.

The whole population is divided into four groups: non-smokers, current smokers, quitters, and those who already suffer from lung cancer. Coefficients describe the risk of lung cancer onset for non-smokers, smokers, and quitters. Transitions between groups are also marked by coefficients.

The population forecast is based on a simplified concept of population dynamics. Using $P_{i,j}(t)$ to denote population at time t, sex i, and age-group j, the equation used is:

$$P_{i,j}(t) = P_{i,j}(t-1) + a - 0.2\,P_{i,j}(t-1) - I_{i,j}\,P_{i,j}(t-1) \qquad i = 1,2 \quad j = 1,\dots,18$$

and if $j = 1$ then a = number of births

$j > 1$ then $a = 0.2\,P_{i,j-1}(t-1)$

$j = 18$ then $P_{i,j}(t-1) = 0$.

The death rate is the total death rate for the population, denoted by I, the mortality rate for non-lung cancer cases is $\tilde{I}$ and lung cancer mortality rate is $\bar{I}$. One can write:

$$I = \tilde{I} + \bar{I} .$$

In order to describe the dynamics of the populations at different risk, we have to introduce some more variables:

$n_{i,j}(t)$ = number of non-smokers with sex i, age j, at time t

$s_{i,j}(t)$ = number of smokers with sex i, age j, at time t

$q_{i,j}(t)$ = number of quitters with sex i, age j, at time t .

Coefficient $p^1_{i,j}$ describes the risk of lung cancer onset for non-smokers with sex i, age j (per 100 000 persons). Coefficients $p^2_{i,j}$ and $p^3_{i,j}$ stand for the same type of risk, but for smokers and quitters, respectively. Transitions between groups are marked by the coefficients $T^1_{i,j}$ for transition from non-smokers to smokers and $T^2_{i,j}$ for transition from smokers to quitters.

One can derive the following equations for the forecast of lung cancer development in non-smokers, smokers, and quitters:

$$n_{i,j}(t) = n_{i,j}(t-1) + a - (T^{1}_{i,j} + c + p^{1}_{i,j} + \tilde{I}_{i,j})\, n_{i,j}(t-1) \qquad i = 1,2 \;\; j = 1,...,18$$

and if $j = 1$ then a = number of births
$j > 1$ then $a = 0.2\, n_{i,j-1}(t-1)$
$j < 18$ then $c = 0.2$
$j, c = 18$ then $c = 0$,

$$s_{i,j}(t) = s_{i,j}(t-1) + a + I^{1}_{i,j}\, n_{i,j}(t) - (p^{2}_{i,j} + c + \tilde{I}_{i,j})\, s_{i,j}(t-1) \qquad i = 1,2 \;\; j = 1,...,18$$

and if $j = 1$ then $a = 0$
$j > 1$ then $a = 0.2\, s_{i,j-1}(t-1)$
$j < 18$ then $c = 0.2$
$j = 18$ then $c = 0$,

$$q_{i,j}(t) = q_{i,j}(t-1) + a + T^{2}_{i,j} s_{i,j}(t) - (p^{3}_{i,j} + c + I_{i,j})\, q_{i,j}(t-1) \qquad i = 1,2 \;\; j = 1,...,18$$

and if $j = 1$ then $a = 0$
$j > 1$ then $a = 0.2\, q_{i,j-1}(t-1)$
$j < 18$ then $c = 0.2$
$j = 18$ then $c = 0$.

The dynamics of lung cancer prevalence, $L_{i,j}(t)$, can be expressed as:

$$L_{i,j}(t) = L_{i,j}(t-1) + p^{1}_{i,j}\; n_{i,j}(t-1) + p^{2}_{i,j} s_{i,j}(t-1) + p^{3}_{i,j}\; q_{i,j}(t-1) + a - (\tilde{I}_{i,j} - \bar{I}_{i,j} + c)\, L_{i,j}(t-1) \qquad i = 1,2 \;\; j = 1,...,18$$

and if $j = 1$ then $a = 0$
$j > 1$ then $a = 0.2\, L_{i,j-1}(t-1)$
$j < 18$ then $c = 0.2$
$j = 18$ then $c = 0$.

Input Data

All input data and results were stratified by sex and age, in 18 age-categories. The initial lung cancer prevalence was estimated from data on lung cancer incidence, according to the following formula:

$$P_{i,j}(t) = 2\, N_{i,j}(t-1) - \bar{I}_{i,j}(t)\, P_{i,j}(t-1)$$

where $P_{i,j}(t)$ stands for lung cancer prevalence at time t, for sex i and age-category j. Lung cancer incidence is represented as $N_{i,j}(t)$ for sex i and age j. Finally, $\bar{I}_{i,j}(t)$ is the lung cancer mortality rate for sex i and age j. All the parameters were stratified over time t.

The input data were identical with those for the DIALOG model described above.

Results

The forecast of male lung cancer morbidity, in five age-groups from 50 to 74 years, is shown in Figure 1. The decrease of morbidity over the years is most pronounced in the older age-groups. The time interval for projections was 12 years, starting in 1985.

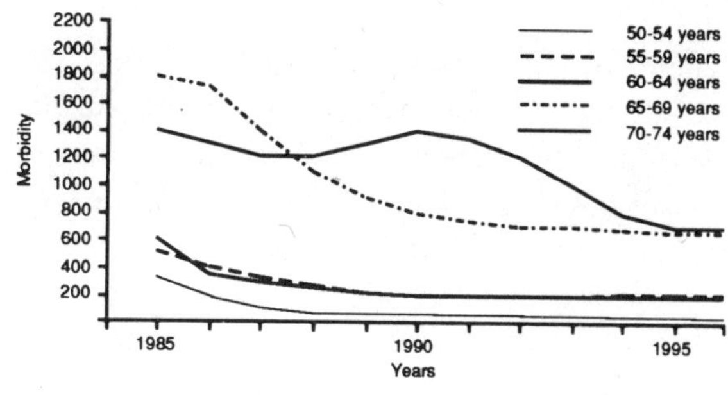

Fig. 1. Lung cancer morbidity forecast for males aged 50-74 years (absolute numbers); basic projection and scenario

Figure 2 depicts data for the female population. The curve is of a different shape, showing a more stable trend compared with the curve for males, suggesting that females are more sensitive than males to risk from smoking. This agrees with the findings from many clinical and epidemiological studies.

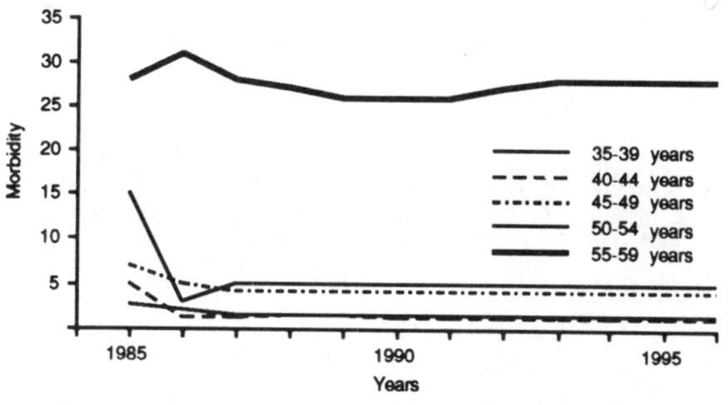

Fig. 2. Lung cancer morbidity forecast for females aged 35-59 years (absolute numbers); basic projection and scenario

Except for the oldest age-group, a decrease in the first two years is followed by a gradual reduction of morbidity with minor fluctuations.

Several scenarios were tested, most of which concerned the situation after a successful anti-smoking campaign. The reduction of smokers was represented by changed values of transition coefficients, namely transitions from smokers to quitters. The other possibility we tested was limitation of risk of smoking, due to the introduction of more efficient cigarette filters or low-tar tobacco. Scenario testing is a primary role for models of this kind, where hypotheses concerning the consequences and efficacy of interventions are being investigated.

Conclusions

The model was run using several scenarios. The original assumption of model sensitivity to minor changes was not proved. However, the results of the model confirmed the general notion that the relationship between smoking and lung cancer is a complex one. It is irrational to expect dramatic changes in smoking behaviour in the developed countries. In addition to public education, several therapeutic methods are used to cure those who wish to stop smoking. Programmes for the early detection of lung cancer, which could improve survival, are very expensive and mass screening is not recommended as a cost-effective measure. This is why smoking cessation may be the only way to stop the increase in lung cancer incidence and mortality.

References

1. Rusnak M, Yashin A, Merinska I (1986) Smoking and Lung Cancer Prevalence: Slovakian Case Study. IIASA, Laxenburg, Collaborative Paper CP-86-12, pp 1-40
2. Scherbov S, Grebucha V (1988) Dial - A System for Modelling Multidimensional Demographic Processes. IIASA, Laxenburg, Working Paper WP-88-36, pp 1-32
3. Katriak M, Javorkova E, Smidtova M (1983) Sociologicke Aspekty Tabakismu. Ustav Zdravotnickej Vychovy, Bratislava, p 97
4. Hammond EC, Percy C (1958) Ex-Smokers. New York State Journal of Medicine (15 September 1958):2956-2959
5. Lubin JH, Bloh WJ, Berrino F, Flamant F, Gillis CR, Kunze M, Schmahl D, Visco G (1984) Modifying risks of developing lung cancer by changing habits of cigarette smoking. Brit Med J 288:1953-1956
6. Enstrom JE (1979) Rising lung cancer mortality among non-smokers. J Nat Cancer Inst 62:755-760
7. Keys A, Menotti A, Aravanis C, Blackburn H, Djordjevic BS, Buzina R, Donpas AS, Sidanza S, Karvonen MJ, Rimura N (1984) The Seven Countries Study: 2.289 deaths in 15 years. Preventive Medicine 13:141-154

Coronary Risk Factors as Predictors of Work Disability and Mortality

M. Heliövaara, A. Rissanen, P. Knekt, A. Reunanen and A. Aromaa

Introduction

Considerable efforts are being made to promote public health awareness and treatment programmes for coronary risk factors, in particular smoking, blood pressure, and serum cholesterol. The substantial contribution of these factors to the incidence of coronary disease, cerebrovascular disease, and cancer has been amply documented in prospective population studies from industrialized countries. From the public health point of view, morbidity leading to premature disability is also an essential outcome criterion in assessing the overall impact of these risk factors. So far, no prospective population studies have focused on this criterion.

The aim of our study was to investigate smoking, body mass index (BMI), diastolic blood pressure, and serum cholesterol level for their prediction of work disability and mortality.

Population and Methods

This study is part of a comprehensive project known as the Social Insurance Institution's *Mobile Clinic Health Examination Survey* [1-5]. The aim of the prospective cohort study was to identify factors predicting disease, and to assess their impact. In 1966-1972, over 57 000 men and women participated in a health examination in various parts of Finland. The 34 study regions, distributed over the whole country, included urban populations, rural populations, and factory employees. The examined groups consisted of either the whole population of a community, or a random sample of it. The participation rate in the survey was 82%. Details of the study population survey methods, and baseline results have been presented previously [1-3].

Baseline health examination by the Mobile Clinic included measurements of height, weight, and blood pressure; ECG; chest X-ray; and biochemical determinations including serum cholesterol level. Information about medical history, occupation, smoking, and other factors was collected using standard questionnaires and interviews.

Morbidity and mortality of all examinees have been followed up continuously. Copies of all death certificates were obtained from the Central Statistical Office of Finland [2]. The study covers the period from the initial examination until 31 December 1982, denoting a mean follow-up of twelve years. The 19 420 women and 22 469 men who were aged 25 or over at the health examination were included in the follow-up analyses. Altogether, 6 766 deaths occurred during 515 230 person-years of follow-up; of these, 3 936 deaths were due to cardiovascular diseases (Table 1).

Table 1. Follow-up experience of the Social Insurance Institution's Health Examination Survey until 31 December 1982

	Women		Men	
	25-64	≥ 65	25-64	≥ 65
Mortality				
Persons	16 919	2 501	20 654	1 815
Person-years	220 832	24 919	254 530	14 949
Deaths, all causes	1 178	1 306	3 007	1 275
Deaths from CVD	615	867	1 718	736
Work disability				
Persons	12 052		19 076	
Person-years	146 839		221 141	
New national invalidity pensions, all	1 710		2 995	
New national invalidity pensions due to CVD	483		1 177	

Data on new national invalidity pensions granted during the follow-up were collected from the Social Insurance Institution's pension register, using a unique personal identification number to link the records. This nationwide register covers data on practically all invalidity pensions. The first day of sick-leave, continued as persistent inability to work, was considered as the beginning of retirement. The primary diagnosis in the doctor's statement for the disability pension was considered as the cause of disability, whatever the disease causing the previous sick-leave. The follow-up experience of work disability refers to the period of observation from the time of the initial examination until early retirement, death, age of 65 years (the general age of retirement in Finland), or the end of the observation period (31 December 1982), whichever came first. Among the *healthy* population of 31 128 women and men, who were in employment and free from perceived work disability at the time of the health examination, 4 705 new invalidity pensions were granted during 367 980 person-years of follow-up; 1 660 of these were due to cardiovascular diseases (Table 1).

An exponential loglinear survival model, an adaptation of the Cox's life-table regression model, was used to analyze the association between the initial levels of risk factors and subsequent morbidity and mortality [6]. The results were expressed as adjusted relative risks (RRs) with 95% confidence intervals (95% CIs), estimated on the basis of the model. The impacts of risk factors on mortality and on incidence of work disability were expressed as *population attributable fractions* [7]. These were calculated on the basis of the adjusted relative risks.

Results

Male smokers aged 25-64 years at entry had a two-fold risk of dying (Table 2), and a two-fold risk of developing work disability (Table 3), as compared with non-smokers. The fractions of mortality and work disability in men attributable to smoking were over 50%, i.e. all-cause mortality and the incidence of work disability in the male population would have been only half of that observed, if the risk for all men had been the risk for those who had never smoked. The impact of smoking was smaller among women (Tables 2 and 3).

In men, daily smoking of 15 cigarettes or more was associated with work disability from cardiovascular (adjusted relative risk, RR = 2.7) and respiratory (RR = 5.1) diseases, as well as from accidental injuries (RR = 3.1) and back pain (RR = 2.1). These rates were highly significant ($p < 0.001$) compared with non-smokers.

In the young and middle-aged (25-64 years at entry) women and men, BMI (weight/height^2) was positively associated with the risk of dying from cardiovascular diseases, but negatively associated with the risk of dying from other diseases combined. The association of BMI with total mortality was weakly U-shaped. Despite its weak association with longevity, BMI was an important predictor of work disability (Table 4), in particular due to cardiovascular diseases and osteoarthritis (data not shown). The fraction of work disability attributable to a BMI exceeding 25 was substantial (27%) in the female population, in which overweight was prevalent, and considerable (7%) among men.

Table 2. Relative risk[1] (RR) and 95% confidence interval (95% CI) of mortality from all causes by smoking history in men and women aged 25-64 at entry

Smoking	%	RR	(95% CI)	Population attributable fraction (%)	
Men					
Never	28.3	1.0			
Stopped	17.6	1.1	(0.8-1.5)	0.3	52.8
Pipe or cigar	4.3	2.2	(1.5-3.1)	4.7	
< 15 cigarettes / day	19.3	1.8	(1.4-2.3)	13.6	
≥ 15 cigarettes / day	30.4	2.7	(2.2-3.4)	34.5	
Women					
Never	80.5	1.0			
Stopped	4.2	1.2	(0.9-1.7)	0.9	8.8
< 15 cigarettes / day	12.6	1.5	(1.3-1.9)	6.4	
≥ 15 cigarettes / day	2.6	2.0	(1.4-2.8)	2.4	

[1] Adjusted for age, area, and body mass index

Elevated diastolic blood pressure was closely associated with the risk of death from cardiovascular diseases, and substantially contributed to total mortality in both the female and male population aged 25-64 at entry. In the fourth and fifth quintiles of diastolic pressure, the relative risks of dying women were 1.4 (95% CI = 1.1-1.6) and 1.8 (1.5-2.1), and in men 1.3 (1.2-1.5) and 1.8 (1.6-2.0), respectively. The fraction of total mortality attributable to these quintiles was 20%. The mortality rates according to systolic pressure followed a similar pattern (data not shown). As expected, elevated blood pressure and medically treated arterial hypertension were highly potent predictors of work disability due to cardiovascular diseases, and contributed also significantly to the total incidence of work disability (Tables 5 and 6).

High levels of serum cholesterol were significantly associated with deaths from cardiovascular diseases in women, and particularly in men aged 25-64 at entry, but seemed to be protective against deaths from other causes. Elevated levels of cholesterol also were associated with disability pensions granted on the

Table 3. Relative risk[1] (RR) and 95% confidence interval (95% CI) of work disability by smoking history in men and women aged 25-64 at entry

Smoking	%	RR	(95% CI)	Population attributable fraction (%)	
Men					
Never	25.8	1.0			
Stopped	21.6	1.4	(1.3-1.6)	8.5	52.5
Pipe or cigar	4.3	2.0	(1.6-2.4)	4.0	
< 15 cigarettes per day	18.6	1.7	(1.5-1.9)	11.5	
≥ 15 cigarettes per day	29.6	2.4	(2.1-2.6)	28.6	
Women					
Never	80.0	1.0			
Stopped	3.9	1.1	(0.8-1.4)	0.3	7.4
< 15 cigarettes per day	13.2	1.5	(1.3-1.7)	6.1	
≥ 15 cigarettes per day	2.8	1.4	(1.0-1.9)	1.1	

[1] Adjusted for age, area, occupation, serum cholesterol, blood pressure, and body mass index

basis of cardiovascular diseases (Table 7), but not with work disability due to other diseases.

In older men (> 65 years at entry), smoking continued to carry a significantly increased risk of dying (1.5-fold total mortality compared with men who had never smoked), but in older women the frequency of smoking was too low to be analyzed for its predictive significance. Diastolic blood pressure was significantly associated with all-cause mortality in the elderly, for both women and men (in the fifth quintiles, RRs = 1.5 and 1.3, respectively), but serum cholesterol and BMI were not.

Discussion

Our cohort represented fairly well the Finnish adult population at large; the distributions of socio-demographic factors and age-specific mortality rates were

Table 4. Relative risk[1] (RR) and 95% confidence interval (95% CI) of work disability by body mass index in men and women aged 25-64 at entry

Body mass index (kg/m^2)	%	RR	(95% CI)	Population attributable fraction (%)	
Men					
< 22.0	14.2	1.0			
22.0 - 24.9	35.1	1.0	(0.9-1.1)		
25.0 - 27.9	31.8	1.1	(1.0-1.2)	2.4	
28.0 - 30.9	14.2	1.2	(1.0-1.4)	2.6	7.1
31.0 - 33.9	3.8	1.3	(1.1-1.6)	1.3	
≥ 34.0	0.9	1.8	(1.3-2.4)	0.8	
Women					
< 22.0	20.2	1.0			
22.0 - 24.9	29.7	1.1	(0.9-1.3)	2.9	
25.0 - 27.9	24.9	1.4	(1.2-1.7)	9.1	
28.0 - 30.9	14.4	1.6	(1.3-1.9)	8.0	27.0
31.0 - 33.9	6.6	1.9	(1.5-2.3)	5.6	
≥ 34.0	4.2	2.1	(1.6-2.6)	4.4	

[1] Adjusted for age, area, occupation, and smoking

very close to those of women and men in the whole country [1, 2]. The follow-up covers all deaths and invalidity pensions. Some generalized conclusions may be warranted about the impact of coronary risk factors, based on the present data. No comparable data are, to our knowledge, available from other countries. Since only modest differences exist between Finland and many industrialized countries with regard to general living conditions and the prevalence of coronary risk factors, the coronary risk factors may have health implications of similar magnitude for other populations. A considerable proportion of morbidity leading to death, and to work disability in particular, could be prevented if the risk factor levels could be modified.

Smoking, a potent risk factor for a number of fatal or disabling diseases, is a major contributor to both disability and premature mortality. However, the

Table 5. Relative risk[1] (RR) and 95% confidence interval (95% CI) of work disability (due to any cause) by blood pressure in men and women aged 25-64 at entry

Blood pressure	%	RR	(95% CI)	Population attributable fraction (%)	
Men					
Normal	45.1	1.0			
Slightly elevated[2]	45.3	1.0	1.0-1.1)	2.1	
Moderately elevated[3]	2.9	1.2	(1.0-1.5)	0.6	5.1
Arterial hypertension[4]	6.8	1.5	(1.3-1.7)	3.0	
Women					
Normal	47.6	1.0			
Slightly elevated[2]	36.8	1.1	(1.0-1.3)	4.2	
Moderately elevated[3]	3.1	1.2	(1.0-1.6)	0.8	10.0
Arterial hypertension[4]	12.5	1.4	(1.2-1.6)	5.0	

[1] Adjusted for age, area, occupation, smoking, body mass index, and serum cholesterol
[2] Systolic > 140 or diastolic > 90
[3] Systolic > 160 and diastolic > 95
[4] Systolic > 170 and diastolic > 100, or anti-hypertensive medication

population-attributable fractions based on our study may be overestimated, as smoking was shown to predict work disability not only from cardiovascular and respiratory diseases, but also from accidental injuries and back pain. These associations suggest indirect and non-causal mechanisms in the relationships, which hamper an assessment of the true preventive potentials.

Elevated levels of blood pressure and serum cholesterol carry substantially increased risks of work disability and death due to cardiovascular diseases. The impact of high blood pressure on public health has previously been described and discussed in detail [1]. But the predictive value of serum cholesterol for all-cause mortality and all-cause disability is limited. The negative association between elevated serum cholesterol levels and non-cardiovascular mortality is mainly due to cancers [8]. However, the increased occurrence of cancer at low cholesterol levels seems to be due to pre-clinical cancer, since the negative as-

Table 6. Relative risk[1] (RR) and 95% confidence interval (95% CI) of work disability due to cardiovascular diseases by blood pressure in men and women aged 25-64 at entry

Blood pressure	%	RR	(95% CI)	Population attributable fraction (%)	
Men					
Normal	45.1	1.0			
Slightly elevated[2]	45.3	1.4	(1.2-1.6)	15.3	29.6
Moderately elevated[3]	2.9	2.2	(1.7-2.8)	3.4	
Arterial hypertension[4]	6.8	2.8	(2.3-3.4)	10.9	
Women					
Normal	47.6	1.0			
Slightly elevated[2]	36.8	1.9	(1.4-2.4)	24.2	54.8
Moderately elevated[3]	3.1	3.0	(2.0-4.6)	5.8	
Arterial hypertension[4]	12.5	3.6	(2.7-4.9)	24.9	

[1] Adjusted for age, area, occupation, smoking, body mass index, and serum cholesterol
[2] Systolic > 140 or diastolic > 90
[3] Systolic > 160 and diastolic > 95
[4] Systolic > 170 and diastolic > 100, or anti-hypertensive medication

sociations are strongest during the first years of follow-up, especially for rapidly developing cancers [8].

Overweight carries an increased risk of work disability and contributes substantially to disability in both sexes, especially in the female population, in which severe overweight is prevalent. Though modest overweight has little impact on longevity [9, 10], it is a major preventable and treatable cause of ill health and disability in affluent populations [5].

To sum up, the coronary risk factors predict both premature mortality and work disability, but through differing disease patterns and with varying power according to age and sex. This should be considered when applying generalized morbidity models to the concept of healthy life expectancy.

Table 7. Relative risk[1] (RR) and 95% confidence interval (95% CI) of work disability due to cardiovascular diseases by serum cholesterol in men and women aged 25-64 at entry

Serum cholesterol (mg/dl)	%	RR	(95% CI)	Population attributable fraction (%)	
Men					
≤ 230	31.4	1.0			
231 - 250	16.0	1.2	(1.0-1.5)	3.1	31.6
251 - 280	22.3	1.4	(1.2-1.7)	7.9	
281 - 310	15.8	1.7	(1.4-1.9)	9.5	
> 310	14.5	1.9	(1.6-2.2)	11.2	
Women					
≤ 230	30.6	1.0			
231 - 250	15.8	1.0	(0.7-1.3)	-0.6	3.9
251 - 280	22.2	0.9	(0.7-1.2)	-2.4	
281 - 310	15.3	1.1	(0.8-1.4)	0.8	
> 310	29.6	1.4	(1.1-1.8)	6.1	

[1] Adjusted for age, area, occupation, smoking, blood pressure, and body mass index

Summary

Smoking, serum cholesterol, blood pressure, and body mass index (kg/m^2) were studied for their prediction of work disability and mortality in a sample of adults from 34 communities in various parts of Finland. In 1966-1972, a total of 41,889 people aged 25 or over (19 420 women and 22 469 men) participated in the Social Insurance Institution's Mobile Clinic Health Examination Survey. Morbidity and mortality of all subjects have been followed up continuously, using record linkage with various registers of health care and social insurance. Data on all deaths and all new national invalidity pensions were obtained up to the end of 1982.

Young and middle-aged (25-64 years at entry) male smokers had a two-fold risk of dying and of developing work disability, as compared with non-smokers. The fractions of mortality and work disability attributable to smoking in the male population of working age were over 50%. The impact of smoking was smaller among women. Body mass index (BMI) had little impact on longevity but was an important predictor of work disability, due in particular to cardiovascular diseases and osteoarthritis. The fraction of work disability attributable to a BMI exceeding 25 was substantial (27%) among women, in whom overweight was prevalent, and considerable (7%) among men. Elevated levels of blood pressure and serum cholesterol were closely associated with the risk of death from cardiovascular diseases and work disability due to cardiovascular diseases, but not due to other diseases. In older people (> 65 years at entry), smoking and blood pressure continued to carry an increased risk of dying, but serum cholesterol and BMI did not.

Coronary risk factors predict both premature mortality and work disability, but through differing disease patterns and with varying power according to age and sex. This should be considered when applying generalized morbidity models to the concept of health life expectancy. A considerable proportion of morbidity leading to death or work disability could be prevented by modifying the risk factor levels.

References

1. Aromaa A (1981) Epidemiology and public health impact of high blood pressure in Finland. Social Insurance Institution, Helsinki
2. Reunanen A, Aromaa A, Pyorala K, Punsar S, Maatela J, Knekt P (1983) The Social Insurance Institution's coronary heart disease study. Baseline data and 5-years mortality experience. Acta Med Scand 214 (Suppl 673)
3. Knekt P (1988) Serum alpha-tokopherol and the risk of cancer. Social Insurance Institution, Helsinki
4. Suhonen O (1988) Sudden coronary death in middle-age in Finland. Publications of the Social Insurance Institution, Helsinki
5. Rissanen A, Heliövaara M, Knekt P, Reunanen A, Aromaa A, Maatela J (1990) Risk of disability and mortality due to overweight in a Finnish population. Med J 301:781-789
6. Kalbfleisch JD, Prentice RL (1980) The statistical analysis of failure time data. Wiley, New York
7. Miettinen OS (1974) Proportion of disease caused or prevented by a given exposure, trait or intervention. Amer J Epidemiol 99:325-332

8. Knekt P, Reunanen A, Aromaa A, Heliövaara M, Hakulinen T, Hakama M (1988) Serum cholesterol and risk of cancer in a cohort of 39 000 men and women. J Clin Epidemiol 41:519-530
9. Rissanen A, Heliövaara M, Knekt P, Aromaa A, Reunanen A, Maatela J (1989) Weight and mortality in Finnish men. J Clin Epidemiol 42:781-789
10. Rissanen A, Knekt P, Heliövaara M, Aromaa A, Reunanen A, Maatela J (1991) Weight and mortality in Finnish women. J Clin Epidemiol (in press)

Longitudinal Models of Disability Changes and Active Life Expectancy in Elderly Populations: The Interaction of Sex, Age and Marital Status

K. G. Manton, E. Stallard and M. A. Woodbury

Introduction

Active life expectancy (ALE) has been used to assess the quality of health and functional changes at advanced ages. By adding a qualitative dimension to life expectancy calculations demographic measures can be made to reflect more closely the social and health service needs of an aging population. This type of measure has been employed for evaluating social and health policy in Japan [1], in France [2], in Canada [3], and recently in the U.S.A. [4].

Although they have clear intuitive appeal, little effort has been expended to develop methodologies for rigorously estimating active life expectancy or to refine the concept. There is still heavy reliance on the basic life table methodology developed for assessing the health of general populations [5].

Several aims have been identified, in order to describe better the health and functional needs of elderly populations. One is to define activity and disability as a graded concept. Past measures have used a simple dichotomy (i.e., disabled or not), which is especially limited when applied to populations of advanced age, in whom there is significant variation in the degree of functional impairment. A second aim is to be able to identify multiple dimensions of functional ability. This is because there are very different social and health policy implications for persons who are cognitively disabled but physically capable, persons who have impaired mobility due to osteoarthritic problems of the lower limbs, and persons who are cognitively intact but who suffer from extreme osteoporosis, which limits all physical activities. Thirdly, one must be able to use longitudinal data to make unbiased estimates of transition rates between *graded* disability states, and of the interaction of disability changes with mortality. Finally, special measurement problems need to be resolved in longitudinal surveys of very elderly persons, especially where non-response is related to serious disability [6].

In this paper we examine how a fuzzy state methodology may be modified to deal with these problems, and illustrate application of the methodology to data from a large national longitudinal survey, the 1982 - 1984 USA National Long Term Care Survey (NLTCS).

Methods

Active Life Expectancy Calculations for Fuzzy States

In order to calculate active life expectancy for individuals, longitudinal information is required on disability changes and on the mortality risks associated with disability. This information can be represented in a two component multivariate stochastic process for cohort [7]. The first component of this process describes the multidimensional changes in disability with age or time, t. The fundamental dynamic equation is

$$g_{it} = C_{t-1}\, g_{i(t-1)} + e_{it} \qquad \text{(i)}$$

where $g_{it} = \{g_{ikt}\}$ are fuzzy state measures of the individual's degree of impairment on each of k =1,..., K functional dimensions at age t; $e_{it} = \{e_{ikt}\}$ are the errors in prediction; $g_{i(t-1)} = \{g_{ik(t-1)}\}$ is the vector of scores at the prior age; and C_{t-1} is the transition matrix. Estimation of the g_{ikt}s is discussed below. See also Manton et al. [8].

In (i) C_{t-1} represents the age dependent matrix of changes in disability status on each of K dimensions between ages t and t-1. Expression (i) represents a system of K equations, where there are constraints on C_{t-1} across equations because the disability scores are constrained such that

$$\sum_k g_{ik} = 1.0 \quad \text{and} \quad 0 \le g_{ik} \le 1.0 \ .$$

The vector of g_{ikt}s represents disability status in terms of its association with K profiles, which are derived from J disability measures, where J>K. The trajectory of the g_{ikt}s over age represents a random walk on a K-1 dimensional simplex defined by K sets of λ_{kjl}s, which are coordinates on the J observed variables.

Since the g_{ikt}s are bounded we cannot directly apply the multivariate Gaussian process described by [7]. Instead the diffusion matrix, which generates the *errors*, e_{ikt}s, in (i), must be generalized to allow changes in the scale of diffusion with age and to reflect boundary restrictions on the fuzzy state space (i.e., the diffusion matrix is scaled by both age and position in the state space). Since λ_{kjl}s which define the state boundaries are generally assumed to be age/time invariant, the trajectories of the g_{ikt}s can be compared at any point in time. A more general model, allowing the λ_{kjl}s to be functions of age(i.e., $\lambda_{kjl(t)}$), has problems of confounding state changes with individual changes in state. Thus, one runs into identifiability problems if λ_{kjl} are allowed to vary.

The second set of equations represents mortality as related to the functional status of persons as indicated on the K fuzzy set scores. This is modelled as a quadratic mortality function which is made age dependent, as,

$$\mu(g_{it}) = (g_{it}^{T}\, Q\, g_{it})\,(\alpha\, e^{\theta t})\,. \tag{ii}$$

In (ii) $\mu(g_{it})$ represents the mortality level which is a quadratic function (where Q contains the quadratic coefficients) of disability status at age t. The g_{ikt}s in (ii) are driven by changes in the dynamics in (i), i.e., mortality changes as a function of the dynamics of the fuzzy disability states. In addition, the Gompertz term, $\alpha e^{\theta t}$ represent the average effects of unknown risk factors associated with age that cause mortality to increase more rapidly than indicated by the disability scores alone, i.e., it represents the average effects of age-related unobserved influential factors. The smaller the value of θ the less is the effect attributed to the *unobserved* variables. If θ is reduced to 0.0, then all age dynamics are described by (i) and the hazard function in (ii) is independent of age.

The coefficients in (i) and (ii) can be introduced into a set of differential equations that represent changes in both disability and mortality by generalized life table functions. The average survival over t to t+1 in a cohort of size l_t is,

$$l_{t+1} = l_t\, |I + V_t\, B_t|^{-1/2} \exp\left\{\frac{\mu_t(\bar{g}_t) + \mu_t(\bar{g}_t^{*})}{2} - 2\,\mu\left(\frac{\bar{g}_t + \bar{g}_t^{*}}{2}\right)\right\} \tag{iii}$$

where $B_t = 1/2\; Q\; e^{\theta t}$, and $\bar{g}_t$ and $\bar{g}_t^{*}$ are the mean g_{ikt}s in the cohort before and after accounting for the mortality effects in (ii), i.e.,

$$\bar{g}_t^{*} = (\bar{g}_t - V_t^{*}\, B_t\, \bar{g}_t) / \sum_k \langle \bar{g}_t - V_t^{*}\, B_t\, \bar{g}_t \rangle_k \tag{iv}$$

where $\langle \cdot \rangle_k$ is the kth element of the enclosed vector, and

$$V_t^{*} = (I + V_t\, B_t)^{-1}\, V_t \tag{v}$$

where V_t is the variance-covariance matrix of the g_{ikt}s.

These parameters are then updated using the dynamics in (i), by

$$\bar{g}_{t+1} = C_t\, \bar{g}_t^{*} \tag{vi}$$

$$V_{t+1} = W_{t+1}\; S\; RS\; W_{t+1} \tag{vii}$$

where R is the sample correlation matrix of the g_{ikt}s after conditioning on age, S is a diagonal matrix with the square roots of the ratios of the variances of the g_{ikt}s to the Bernoulli bounds on its diagonal, and W^2_{t+1} is a diagonal matrix of Bernoulli bounds where $w^2_{kk(t+1)} = \bar{g}_{k(t+1)} \cdot (1 - \bar{g}_{k(t+1)})$.

Identification of Fuzzy States

Equations (iii) - (vii) can be used to construct fuzzy state specific life tables. The g_{ikt}s are latent variables estimated from GoM, a fuzzy set multivariate procedure [9]. This procedure uses maximum likelihood (ML) procedures to estimate

$$\Pr(y_{ijl} = 1.0) = \sum_k g_{ik} \lambda_{kjl} \qquad \text{(viii)}$$

where y_{ijl} is a 0-1 binary variable obtained from a data matrix $\{x_{ij}\}$ for i = 1,..., I cases (persons) and j = 1,..., J variables using $y_{ijl} = 1$ if $x_{ij} = l$, where l=1,..., L_j are discrete responses.

The λ_{kjl}s are the basis for constructing the simplex in the J variable measurement space within which the g_{ik}s are constrained.

To apply the methodology to longitudinal national survey data two additional factors need to be taken into account. One is the effect of complex sample design. This is handled by realizing that (a) the λ_{kjl}s are estimated conditional upon their own set of individual specific state variables (g_{ikt}), and (b) since this produces appropriate MLEs for the λ_{kjl}s it remains only to adjust the g_{ikt}s by post-weighting for their sample selection probability [8].

Response rates vary as a function of health and functional status. Thus, we can expect bias in the estimates. To make informed adjustments to the g_{ikt}s we used ML procedures. Specifically, because in the NLTCS we have a list sample drawn from Medicare administrative records, we know the vital status for every person, respondent or not. For respondents we can, within age- and sex-specific cells, estimate the mortality function for the estimated g_{ikt} values. Thus, for non-respondents we can calculate the mortality rates assuming that the age- and sex-specific rates for respondents applied. If the predicted mortality rate is different from the one observed, this suggests that the g_{ikt} distribution is different for non-respondents than for respondents in the same cell. The ML procedures indicate how the g_{ikt} distribution for non-respondents should be altered [8]. This will tell us how to re-normalize the weights for respondents to correctly adjust the g_{ikt} distribution for non-response bias.

Morbidity Changes and Fuzzy State Systems and their Respondence

One may wish to simulate changes in the age-dependent multivariate disablement process due to morbidity onset, changes in social status, or some other aspect of behaviour. One approach is to realize that the moments of the g_{ik} parameters are consistently estimable [10], and that the g_{ikt} distribution can be used in subsequent statistical analyses and simulations. This provides a way of estimating how disability would be altered if, for example, morbidity were changed. Specifically, we can estimate how the distribution of disability would be affected if certain statuses or conditions were eliminated.

This is done in two stages. First we determine how the initial distribution of the g_{ikt}s at age t_0, is altered. Second, we determine how the transition matrix C_t in (i) and (vi) is altered.

Let m=1,..., M denote the classes of a discrete variable D, such that $D_{im} = 1$ implies that individual i is in Class m. Let p_{mt} be the age specific probability that $D_{im} = 1$, independent of i. Then

$$\bar{g}_{kt} = \sum_{m} p_{mt}\, \bar{g}_{kt}^{(m)} \qquad \text{(ix)}$$

where $\bar{g}_{kt}^{(m)}$ is the conditional mean of g_{ikt}, given that $D_{im} = 1$. The elimination of Class m from the population yields the altered mean

$$\bar{g}_{kt}^{(\bar{m})} = \sum_{n \neq m} p_{nt}\, \bar{g}_{kt}^{(n)} / \sum_{n \neq m} p_{nt} \qquad \text{(x)}$$

which may be used to determine the initial cohort mean g_{ikt}s at age $t = t_0$.

To compute the transition matrix $C_t = \{c_{klt}\}$ in (i), we define g_{iklt} as the joint membership in Classes k and *l* of the GoM model at ages t and t+1 respectively. Following Manton et al. [8], let

$$c_{klt} = \bar{g}_{klt} / \bar{g}_{kt} \qquad \text{(xi)}$$

where $\bar{g}_{klt}$ is the age-specific mean of g_{iklt}. Letting $\bar{g}_{klt}^{(m)}$ be the conditional mean, given $D_{im} = 1$, we have

$$\bar{g}_{klt} = \sum_{m} p_{mt}\, \bar{g}_{klt}^{(m)} \qquad \text{(xii)}$$

and upon elimination of Class m from the population:

$$\bar{g}_{klt}^{(\bar{m})} = \sum_{n \neq m} p_{nt}\, \bar{g}_{klt}^{(n)} \Big/ \sum_{n \neq m} p_{nt} \,. \tag{xiii}$$

Hence

$$c_{klt}^{(\bar{m})} = \bar{g}_{klt}^{(\bar{m})} / \bar{g}_{kt}^{(\bar{m})} = \sum_{n \neq m} p_{nt}\, \bar{g}_{klt}^{(n)} \Big/ \sum_{n \neq m} p_{nt}\, \bar{g}_{kt}^{(n)} \,. \tag{xiv}$$

Defining $C_t^{(\bar{m})} = \{c_{klt}^{(\bar{m})}\}$, we can replace C_t in (vi) to obtain a modified cohort life table consistent with (x).

This is done in the example to generate life tables specific to the marital status categories, married and non-married. In this example, however, we also estimated Q_t stratified by marital status, so that the entire analysis separated into two independent components. This was done because the presence of a spouse could have a direct effect on reducing mortality risks, as well as indirect effects on mortality through C_t.

More generally, instead of D_{im} (a discrete indicator of whether the person had the mth status or condition) we could estimate S_{iw}, a set of W fuzzy set scores independently estimated from J^* social (or other) variables, where $W < J^*$. Suppose we estimated S_{iw} from a GoM analysis of income, education, living arrangements, marital status, family size, etc. Then we would relate the W dimensions that describe those measures to disability as

$$\bar{g}_{kt} = \sum_{w} \bar{S}_{wt}\, \bar{g}_{kt}^{(w)} \tag{xv}$$

where $\bar{S}_{wt}$ is the mean of S_{iw} at age t and $\bar{g}_{kt}^{(w)}$ the conditional mean of g_{ikt}, given that $S_{iw} = 1$. Similarly,

$$\bar{g}_{klt} = \sum_{w} \bar{S}_{wt}\, \bar{g}_{klt}^{(w)} \tag{xvi}$$

where the ratio (xvi) to (xv) yields c_{klt} as in (xi).

In this case the transition matrix C_t is parameterized through $\bar{S}_{wt}$ as a function of social as well as medical diagnoses and other variables. This reduces the parameterization to the information in $\bar{S}_{wt}$, so that an intervention is modelled by specifying how $\bar{S}_{wt}$ changes. In the case that one component of a dichotomous variable is deleted, one need only recompute the mean S_{iw}s for the retained component, replacing $\bar{S}_{wt}$ in (xv) and (xvi). More generally, these forms of equations can be used to embed multiple fuzzy state representations of relevant subsystems in simulation and forecasting procedures in a way that is both dimensionally parsimonious and restricted to a metric that is natural for describing discrete attributes.

Data

The data used are drawn from the 1982-1984 NLTCS. This survey of elderly Medicare recipients is drawn from a list sample which allows tracking mortality and Medicare service use of *all* persons in the sample - *including* non-respondents. The disability dimensions were determined from 27 functional measures. From the 27 measures, 6 fuzzy classes were formed which can be described as follows [6]:

1. Nonchronical functionally impaired
2. Functionally intact with instrumental activities of daily living (IADL) associated with cognitive functioning
3. Limited IADL limitation and moderate physical impairment
4. High degrees of physical impairment and some IADL impairment
5. Frail elderly (i.e., moderate ADL impairment) but no cognitive limitation
6. Highly impaired in ADL, IADL and physical functioning.

A seventh *discrete* class was assigned to institutional members of the list sample $g_{i7} = 1$, else $g_{i7} = 0$. Medicare administrative records identified mortality for both the 1982 and 1984 samples for two years after the end of the survey period (i.e., a total four-year period, 1982 to 1986).

Results

Results are presented for ALE, for married and unmarried US males and females. There is literature on marital status differences in mortality in the USA [11] but marital status has never before been linked longitudinally to detailed disablement processes.

Disability Dynamics: Age and Marital State Specific Fuzzy State Transitions

Two types of matrices are required to calculate ALE from (iii) to (vii). The first are transition matrices, which are functions of marital status (and could be made functions of other domains of interest) and age. These matrices, evaluated at age 75, are presented in Table 1 and Table 2.

In the male table there is a large difference (9%) in the likelihood of remaining healthy for two more years at age 75 between married (95%) and unmarried (86%) males. The majority of unmarried males who lose their active status go to Class 5 (frail with multiple pulmonary and cardiovascular problems) and into institutions. For Classes 2 and 5, the likelihood of remaining independent was preserved equally well for married and unmarried males. The risk of going to institutions in most classes (but not Class 1 or 5) is slightly *higher* for married males. For Classes 3, 4, and 6, institutionalized unmarried males are more likely to return to a healthy state. Thus, if initially *healthy*, married males are more likely to remain so than unmarried males. If in a disabled state, however, unmarried males are more likely to return to a healthy state. This is because *married* males have higher survival rates in impaired states.

Married females are a little more likely to remain healthy than are unmarried females. In contrast to males, *married* females are more likely to return to a nondisabled state at all levels of impairment. Likewise, the likelihood of institutionalization is also reversed, with *unmarried* females more likely to be institutionalized.

The age dependence of the transition matrices is shown in Table 3, which contains two-year transitions for persons starting in the healthy class at ages 65, 75, 85, and 95.

There is little difference for married and unmarried females in the age-specific transitions, though there is a decline in the proportion that remain healthy over two years, and large increases in persons in institutions and in most disabled states.

Married males, in contrast, show a greater likelihood of remaining active over two years than unmarried males - a preservation of functional ability is maintained at all ages. Unmarried males end up with higher rates of institutionalization.

Table 1. Male specific disability state transitions evaluated for married and unmarried persons at age 75[1]

Class at time 1	Class at time 2 1 Healthy	2 Early cognitive impairment	3 Moderate physical impairment	4 Heavy physical impairment	5 Frail	6 Highly impaired	Institution-alized
1 Healthy							
Married	0.950	0.009	0.008	0.003	0.011	0.013	0.006
Unmarried	0.864	0.013	0.008	0.010	0.039	0.018	0.049
2 Early cognitive impairment							
Married	0.500	0.190	0.099	0.024	0.061	0.094	0.034
Unmarried	0.500	0.184	0.040	0.057	0.076	0.144	0.0
3 Moderate physical impairment							
Married	0.411	0.092	0.098	0.059	0.161	0.086	0.093
Unmarried	0.489	0.031	0.081	0.015	0.258	0.092	0.032
4 Heavy physical impairment							
Married	0.263	0.074	0.071	0.145	0.210	0.142	0.092
Unmarried	0.483	0.100	0.033	0.043	0.172	0.081	0.088
5 Frail							
Married	0.518	0.047	0.049	0.052	0.176	0.126	0.031
Unmarried	0.525	0.001	0.027	0.053	0.281	0.058	0.056
6 Highly impaired							
Married	0.338	0.049	0.033	0.034	0.049	0.374	0.124
Unmarried	0.488	0.014	0.033	0.029	0.123	0.234	0.080
Institutionalized							
Married	0.212	0.003	0.0	0.0	0.016	0.0	0.770
Unmarried	0.246	0.009	0.022	0.011	0.059	0.0	0.654

[1] Source: 1982 - 1984 National Long Term Care Survey

Table 2. Female specific disability state transitions evaluated for married and unmarried persons at age 75[1]

Class at time 1	Class at time 2 1 Healthy	2 Early cognitive impairment	3 Moderate physical impairment	4 Heavy physical impairment	5 Frail	6 Highly impaired	Institution-alized
1 Healthy							
Married	0.927	0.008	0.011	0.038	0.018	0.013	0.018
Unmarried	0.919	0.013	0.016	0.011	0.019	0.009	0.013
2 Early cognitive impairment							
Married	0.478	0.067	0.059	0.066	0.140	0.131	0.059
Unmarried	0.372	0.130	0.079	0.053	0.107	0.059	0.201
3 Moderate physical impairment							
Married	0.500	0.057	0.132	0.090	0.123	0.074	0.023
Unmarried	0.447	0.053	0.125	0.093	0.094	0.075	0.114
4 Heavy physical impairment							
Married	0.541	0.079	0.051	0.075	0.074	0.158	0.023
Unmarried	0.458	0.030	0.083	0.147	0.065	0.117	0.100
5 Frail							
Married	0.406	0.042	0.117	0.088	0.250	0.089	0.008
Unmarried	0.399	0.051	0.075	0.069	0.272	0.079	0.055
6 Highly impaired							
Married	0.446	0.070	0.076	0.189	0.057	0.134	0.028
Unmarried	0.279	0.058	0.045	0.074	0.118	0.303	0.123
Institutionalized							
Married	0.344	0.0	0.0	0.082	0.0	0.002	0.573
Unmarried	0.184	0.010	0.018	0.017	0.023	0.010	0.732

[1]Source: 1982 - 1984 National Long Term Care Survey

Table 3. Two-year transitions for married and unmarried persons who were initially healthy at ages 65, 75, 85, and 95[1]

Age	Class 1 Healthy	2 Early cognitive impairment	3 Moderate physical impairment	4 Heavy physical impairment	5 Frail	6 Highly impaired	Institution-alized
				Unmarried females			
65	0.932	0.010	0.022	0.007	0.015	0.007	0.008
75	0.919	0.013	0.016	0.014	0.019	0.009	0.013
85	0.771	0.039	0.032	0.024	0.043	0.022	0.064
95	0.680	0.085	0.036	0.015	0.055	0.042	0.086
				Married females			
65	0.966	0.002	0.012	0.004	0.007	0.009	0.001
75	0.927	0.008	0.011	0.004	0.018	0.013	0.018
85	0.782	0.060	0.022	0.013	0.063	0.027	0.033
95	0.633	0.052	0.0	0.013	0.204	0.0	0.097
				Unmarried males			
65	0.951	0.014	0.002	0.001	0.022	0.006	0.003
75	0.864	0.011	0.008	0.010	0.004	0.018	0.049
85	0.794	0.023	0.021	0.001	0.073	0.034	0.055
95	0.734	0.063	0.026	0.008	0.053	0.043	0.073
				Married males			
65	0.956	0.005	0.013	0.005	0.009	0.012	0.0
75	0.950	0.009	0.008	0.003	0.011	0.013	0.006
85	0.870	0.029	0.013	0.004	0.035	0.026	0.023
95	0.785	0.039	0.022	0.012	0.043	0.061	0.037

[1] Source: 1982 - 1984 National Long Term Care Survey

Mortality Functions

The second set of matrices are the quadratic mortality functions. The coefficients from the matrix Q evaluated at age 75, are presented in Tables 4 and 5. Since the matrices are symmetric, we present only the upper half (including the diagonal).

In these tables, the coefficients along the diagonal represent the annual mortality rate for a person who fits exactly into a class. Suppose, however, that a person is a partial member of two classes (e.g., $g_{i4} = 0.5$ and $g_{i6} = 0.5$). Then one would calculate a mortality rate of

$$\mu(g_{ik}) = [\{(-0.061) \times 2\} \cdot 0.5^2] + 0.004 \cdot 0.5^2 + 0.987 \cdot 0.5^2 = 0.217$$

for unmarried males. The negative values for unmarried males in Class 4 suggest that living in that class moderately reduces mortality for someone who is a partial member of one or more other classes. This is a function of the short time a person is expected to spend in that class (i.e., his two-year retention is only 4.3%).

Mortality coefficients are higher for unmarried than married males. This is most evident for Classes 1, 2, 5 and 6. The coefficients are age-dependent because their effects increase as a Gompertz function of age. The Gompertz coefficient, θ, indicates that risks increase more rapidly with age for married than for unmarried males, i.e., 4.04% versus 3.27% per year of age. Thus, the survival advantages of married males are concentrated at younger ages. Mortality for unmarried males is extremely high for Class 6 (i.e., 62.7%/year = $1 - e^{-0.987}$ at age 75). Thus, for Class 6 social inputs seem to help reduce mortality.

For females there is less difference in mortality with marital status. The θ parameters governing age increases in mortality are nearly identical for differences in marital status (i.e., 3.67% versus 3.59%). The differences in the Q coefficients are less than for males.

Overall, the size of the Gompertz parameters (3.3% to 4.0%) are much smaller than when estimated from mortality data with no covariates (usually 8% - 10%). Thus, the disability dynamics explain much of the age dependency of mortality. If functional status can be preserved, age-specific mortality rates can be greatly reduced.

Table 4. Quadratic mortality functions evaluated for males at age 75

Class	1 Healthy	2 Early cognitive impairment	3 Moderate physical impairment	4 Heavy physical impairment	5 Frail	6 Highly impaired	Institution-alized
1 Healthy							
Married (θ=0.0404)	0.034	0.058	0.082	0.016	0.057	0.141	0.090
Unmarried (θ=0.0327)	0.050	0.074	0.097	-0.014	0.080	0.223	0.108
2 Early Cognitive impairment							
Married		0.099	0.139	0.027	0.098	0.241	0.153
Unmarried		0.109	0.142	-0.020	0.118	0.327	0.158
3 Moderate physical impairment							
Married			0.195	0.038	0.137	0.337	0.214
Unmarried			0.186	-0.027	0.155	0.429	0.207
4 Heavy physical impairment							
Married				0.007	0.027	0.066	0.042
Unmarried				0.004	-0.022	-0.061	-0.030
5 Frail							
Married					0.097	0.238	0.151
Unmarried					0.128	0.356	0.172
6 Highly impaired							
Married						0.585	0.371
Unmarried						0.987	0.477
Institutionalized							
Married							0.235
Unmarried							0.231

Table 5. Quadratic mortality functions evaluated for females at age 75

Class	1 Healthy	2 Early cognitive impairment	3 Moderate physical impairment	4 Heavy physical impairment	5 Frail	6 Highly impaired	Institution-alized
1 Healthy							
Married (θ=0.0367)	0.017	0.044	0.030	0.009	0.031	0.079	0.061
Unmarried (θ=0.0359)	0.021	0.038	0.027	0.022	0.034	0.085	0.056
2 Early cognitive impairment							
Married		0.111	0.075	0.024	0.078	0.198	0.154
Unmarried		0.069	0.050	0.040	0.062	0.155	0.102
3 Moderate physical impairment							
Married			0.050	0.016	0.053	0.134	0.104
Unmarried			0.036	0.029	0.045	0.113	0.074
4 Heavy physical impairment							
Married				0.005	0.017	0.043	0.033
Unmarried				0.023	0.036	0.090	0.060
5 Frail							
Married					0.056	0.141	0.019
Unmarried					0.055	0.140	0.092
6 Highly impaired							
Married						0.355	0.275
Unmarried						0.351	0.231
Institutionalized							
Married							0.213
Unmarried							0.152

Active Life Expectancy Estimates

With the mortality and transition matrices (age and marital status dependent) we can construct disability-specific life tables. The matrices show that much of the differential in disability over marital status for males comes from mortality differentials. For females, mortality differences are small, but the disability transition matrices show significant differences. Thus, there is an essential difference in the dynamics driving disability in elderly males and females, which are likely to have their basis in latent multidimensional physiological processes correlated with functional changes.

In Table 6 we present the life expectancy in specific disability states for ages 65, 75, 85, and 95, for married and unmarried males.

At age 65, marital status has a 3.5 year effect on male total life expectancy, and a 3.8 year effect on male ALE. Married males have longer life expectancies in Classes 2, 3, and 6. The expected time in institutions is higher (0.69 versus 0.33 years) for unmarried males at age 65. The smaller expected time in Class 6 for unmarried males suggests that the presence of a spouse allows a male to stay out of institutions even at that high level of frailty. Why unmarried males should have a greater prevalence in Classes 4 and 5 is less clear. It may be that marital status reduces risks of cardiopulmonary and joint conditions, which increase the risk of entering these classes.

At age 85 the difference in life expectancy due to marital status is only 1.1 years, i.e., it has declined faster than total life expectancy. Thus, the positive effect of marital status on male survival is more strongly manifest at younger ages -- this is consistent with the higher θ for married males. The difference in ALE is 1.4 years so that there is an additional benefit of being married in maintaining functional status, e.g., at age 65, 89% of life expectancy is expected to be active for married males compared to 83% for unmarried males. The relative difference is larger at age 85, when it is 75% versus 65%. The difference in expected time in an institution remains nearly the same (i.e., 0.72 years for unmarried versus 0.43 for married). Likewise, Class 6, at age 85, has a very similar life expectancy to that at age 65. This is because of the high-risk nature of Class 6, which dominates the average effect on mortality. Female results are also presented in Table 6 for ages 65, 75, 85, and 95.

The differential in total life expectancy at age 65 due to marital status is less than for males (i.e., 0.6 years versus 3.5 years). The increase in ALE is greater (i.e., 1.7 years or 83% versus 78%) due to a shorter expected time in institutions (i.e., married women can expect to spend 0.83 years in institutions, as compared to 1.5 years for unmarried women). This is manifest, as for men, in a higher prevalence of Class 6 women in the married group.

Table 6. Life expectancy at ages 65, 75, 85, and 95

Age	Total	Class 1 Healthy	2 Early cognitive impairment	3 Moderate physical impairment	4 Heavy physical impairment	5 Frail	6 Highly impaired	Institution-alized
				Males				
65								
Married	16.37	14.53	0.301	0.243	0.143	0.367	0.467	0.328
Unmarried	12.91	10.75	0.267	0.175	0.155	0.559	0.314	0.686
75								
Married	11.50	9.71	0.330	0.196	0.119	0.324	0.461	0.359
Unmarried	9.12	6.98	0.283	0.150	0.132	0.499	0.314	0.753
85								
Married	7.09	5.33	0.311	0.166	0.092	0.300	0.468	0.430
Unmarried	5.95	3.89	0.328	0.154	0.078	0.482	0.299	0.715
95								
Married	4.60	3.23	0.221	0.118	0.072	0.210	0.398	0.353
Unmarried	4.25	2.59	0.291	0.121	0.052	0.344	0.252	0.600
				Females				
65								
Married	20.67	17.16	0.434	0.423	0.345	0.748	0.736	0.830
Unmarried	20.10	15.64	0.576	0.587	0.464	0.734	0.586	1.511
75								
Married	14.17	10.82	0.439	0.305	0.265	0.714	0.714	0.913
Unmarried	13.93	9.64	0.568	0.464	0.379	0.669	0.584	1.629
85								
Married	8.10	5.00	0.404	0.185	0.160	0.640	0.738	0.970
Unmarried	8.49	4.61	0.514	0.358	0.278	0.513	0.563	1.658
95								
Married	4.40	1.85	0.329	0.040	0.103	0.571	0.340	1.167
Unmarried	5.58	2.61	0.457	0.236	0.182	0.326	0.503	1.262

At age 85 there is a small (0.4 years) advantage for unmarried women, i.e., the advantage became reversed between age 83 and 84. Nonetheless, the proportion of life expected to be active remained higher - 62% versus 54%. Married women still stayed out of institutions 0.7 years longer, which was reflected in a higher prevalence of Classes 5 and 6 for married women. Thus, the patterns at age 85 are different for men and women.

Summary

We used fuzzy state methods to define disability states, which were used to calculate measures of active and disabled life expectancy specific to sex, age and marital status. For males, there were large differences in the effects of marital status on both total life expectancy and ALE. For females, the effects on total life expectancy were smaller than for males, but there was a significant effect on ALE.

The mechanisms causing the effects of marital status on survival were very different for males and females. Marital status had a large effect on mortality for males, while it had more effect on disability transitions for females. Thus, the mechanisms determining the interaction of marital status, age and disablement varied by sex.

We have shown the calculations for the effects of marital status. However, the results could be generalized to cases where multidimensional fuzzy state systems interact. The fuzzy state representation thus offers a flexible way of representing the interactions of complex multidimensional systems in forecasting human survival and health changes at advanced ages.

Acknowledgements

This research was supported by NIA grants 5R37AG07198, 5R37AG07025, 1R01AG07469, 5R01AG01159, and 2R37AG03188; and HCFA grant 18-C-98641/4-03S2.

References

1. Nihon University (1982) Population Aging in Japan: Problems and Policy Issues in the 21st Century. In: Kuroda T (ed) International Conference on an Aging Society: Strategies for 21st Century Japan (Nihon University, Japan, Nov. 1982). Nihon University Population Research Institute, Tokyo

2. Robine JM, Labbe M, Serouss MC, Colvez A (1989) The Upper-Normandy Longitudinal Survey on Disability in the Aged, 1978-1985. Revue d'Epidemiologie et de Sante Publique 37 (1):37-48
3. Wilkins R, Adams O (1983) Healthfulness of Life. Institute for Research on Public Policy, Montreal
4. Crimmins E, Saito Y, Ingegneri D (1989) Changes in life expectancy and disability-free life expectancy in the United States. Population and Development Review 15:235-267
5. Sullivan DF (1971) A single index of mortality and morbidity. HSMHA Health Reports 86:347-354
6. Manton KG, Stallard E (1991) Cross-sectional estimates of active life expectancy for the U.S. elderly and oldest-old populations. Journal of Gerontology 48:170-182
7. Woodbury MA, Manton KG (1983) A theoretical model of the physiological dynamics of circulatory disease in human populations. Human Biology 55:417-441
8. Manton KG, Woodbury MA, Corder LS, Stallard E (1992) The use of Grade of Membership to estimate regression relationships. In: Marsden P (ed) Sociological Methodology 1992. (in press)
9. Woodbury MA Clive J, Garson A (1978) Mathematical typology: A grade of membership technique for obtaining disease definition. Computers and Biomedical Research 11:277-298
10. Tolley HD, Manton KG (1991) Large sample properties of a fuzzy partition. Journal of Statistical Mathematics (in press)
11. Retherford RD (1975) The Changing Sex Differential in Mortality. Greenwood Press, Westport

Competing Risks Modelling in Contaminated Populations

A. I. Michalski

Problem Statement

The basic assumption of competing risks modelling deals with probabilistic relations between risks. The assumption of independent risks is used more frequently than that of dependent risks. The reason for this is that in the case of independent risks the calculations of the survival function, death rate, morbidity and other related functions may be made only on the basis of information about the population.

The case of dependent risks requires additional information on the nature of the risks dependency. An example of such approach can be found in [1]. The authors consider competing risks that are conditionally independent of the trajectory of a stochastic process $\mathbf{Z}_t$. In this case the conditional survival function may be written in the form:

$$S(t \mid \mathbf{Z}_t) = e^{-\int_0^t \sum_{i=1}^k \mu_i(\tau, \mathbf{Z}_t)\, d\tau}$$

where $\mu_i(\tau, \mathbf{Z}_t)$ is the mortality rate due to the ith cause of death conditioned on the trajectory $\mathbf{Z}_t$. The unconditional survival function $S(t)$ in this case has a form

$$S(t) = e^{-\int_0^t \bar{\mu}(\tau)\, d\tau}$$

where $(\tau) = E\left(\int_0^t \sum_{i=1}^k \mu_i(\tau, \mathbf{Z}_t)\, d\tau\right)$ is the expectation of the total mortality rate over the process $\mathbf{Z}_t$.

The problem is how to calculate the expectation $\bar{\mu}(\tau)$. In [1] some formulas for $\bar{\mu}(\tau)$ derived for the following specific case. The mortality rate due to a specific cause of death $\mu_i(\tau, \mathbf{Z}_t)$ is a quadratic function on $\mathbf{Z}_t$:

$$\mu_i(\tau, \mathbf{Z}_t) = \tilde{\mu}_i(\tau)\, \mathbf{Z}_t^2$$

where $\tilde{\mu}_i(\tau)$ are age-dependent mortality rates and the process $\mathbf{Z}_t$ satisfies a linear diffusion type stochastic differential equation:

$$d\mathbf{Z}_t = (a_0(t) + a_1(t)\, \mathbf{Z}_t)\, dt + \beta(t)\, dW_t\,, \quad \mathbf{Z}_0 = z_o\ .$$

The expectation of the mortality rate in this case has the form

$$\mu(\tau) = m^2(\tau) + \gamma(\tau)$$

where $m(\tau)$ and $\gamma(\tau)$ satisfy the nonlinear ordinary differential equations

$$m(\tau) = \alpha_0(\tau) + \alpha_1(\tau)\, m(\tau) - 2\gamma(\tau) \sum_{i=1}^{k} \tilde{\mu}_i(\tau)$$

$$\gamma(\tau) = 2\alpha_1(\tau)\, \gamma(\tau) + \beta^2(\tau) - 2\gamma^2(\tau) \sum_{i=1}^{k} \tilde{\mu}_i(\tau)\ .$$

The identification of functions $\alpha_0(\tau)$, $\alpha_1(\tau)$ and $\beta(\tau)$ and initial conditions require much preliminary and experimental information. There are many cases where such information is not available and different approaches must be used.

The other approach to dependent competing risks analysis is to consider two populations. One, say a *pure population*, may be considered as a population with independent competing risks. The other, say a *contaminated population*, is to be considered as a population with dependent risks. The interpretation of this situation is obvious. The *pure population* may represent residents of an ecologically safe region, the *contaminated population* may represent residents of a region with bad ecological conditions. The environmental pollution will act on the *pure population* changing people's resistance to different risk factors, and in time, will lead the population to the state of the *contaminated population*. Using *pure* population data one can extract information which can be used to compensate for the lack of information on dependent risk case.

In this paper we consider a mathematical description of the dependent competing risks problem. We describe concomitant mathematical problems and discuss ways of their solution.

Mathematical Description

It is reasonable to describe the negative influence of environmental pollution in terms of a risk factor which leads to an increase in the rates of cause-specific mortality. We assume that the proportion of individual increase in each cause-specific mortality rate has the same value for different causes of death. The value of the proportion varies from individual to individual and we consider it to be the random variable. The physiological explanation of the risk factor may be human frailty due to environmental pollution. Assumptions made lead to the proportional dependent risk model (PDRM).

Let $\mu_j(t)$ denote net mortality rate due to cause of death j (j = 1, ..., k). They are rates in the *pure population.* Let β denote the value of a risk factor acting on the individual mortality rate. The net individual mortality rate due to cause j in a *contaminated population* equals $\beta\mu_j(t)$. The aggregate mortality rate for a person is given by the expression

$$\mu(t,\beta) = \beta \sum_{i=1}^{k} \mu_i(t) \ .$$

The joint survival function in the *contaminated population* is a mean value of the individual cause-specific survival functions product

$$S(t_1, ..., t_k) = \int e^{-\beta \sum_{i=1}^{k} \int_0^{t_i} \mu_i(\tau)\, d\tau} dP(\beta)$$

where $P(\beta)$ is the probability distribution function of factor β.

The crude cause-specific mortality rate may then be expressed in the form

$$\hat{\mu}_j(t) = \frac{-\frac{\partial}{\partial t_j} S(t_1, ..., t_k) \mid_{t_1 = ... t_k = t}}{S(t_1, ..., t_k)} = \mu_j(t)\, K\Big(\sum_{i=1}^{k} \int_0^t \mu_i(\tau)\, d\tau \Big) \qquad (1)$$

where

$$K(a) = \frac{\int \beta\, e^{-a\beta}\, dP(\beta)}{\int e^{-a\beta}\, dP(\beta)} \ .$$

Illustrative Example

To illustrate relation (1) we consider a simple example of probability distribution $P(\beta)$. Define $P(\beta)$ as follows:

$$P(\beta) = 0 \qquad \text{if } \beta < 1$$
$$P(\beta) = 1 - e^{-\lambda\beta} \qquad \text{if } \beta \geq 1 .$$

This distribution relates to the case of a heterogeneous population with parameter β exponentially distributed from 1 to infinity. It models the negative influence of environmental contamination on population health. The value of parameter λ shows the degree of heterogeneity in population. The less λ the more heterogeneous is the population. When λ tends to 0 the population tends to the homogeneous one.

The value of the crude cause-specific mortality rate gives the formula

$$\hat{\mu}_j(t) = \mu_j(t) \left(1 + \left(\lambda + \sum_{i=1}^{k} \int_0^t \mu_i(\tau)\, d\tau \right)^{-1} \right)$$

and the survival function in the heterogeneous population is

$$S(t) = e^{-\int_0^t \sum_{i=1}^{k} \hat{\mu}_i(\tau)\, d\tau}$$
$$= e^{-\int_0^t \sum_{i=1}^{k} \mu_i(\tau)\, d\tau}\; e^{-\sum_{i=1}^{k} \int_0^t \mu_i(\tau) \left(\lambda + \sum_{j=1}^{k} \int_0^\tau \mu_j(\xi)\, d\xi \right)^{-1} d\tau} .$$

The cause-elimination survival function is

$$\hat{S}_{\bullet r}(t) = e^{-\int_0^t \sum_{i=1, i\neq r}^{k} \mu_i(\tau)\, d\tau}\; e^{-\sum_{i=1, i\neq r}^{k} \int_0^t \mu_i(\tau) \left(\lambda + \sum_{j=1, j\neq r}^{k} \int_0^\tau \mu_j(\xi)\, d\xi \right)^{-1} d\tau} .$$

Real Population Study

There are two main problems in proportional conditionally independent competing risk analysis:

- how to estimate probability distribution function $P(\beta)$, and
- how to estimate the cause-elimination survival function $\hat{S}_{\bullet r}(t)$ when net mortality rates $\mu_i(t)$ are unknown?

These problems may be solved on the basis of cause-specific mortality data in a *pure population*. In this part we consider how to use this information for the estimation of distribution function $P(\beta)$.

Let $\hat{S}_i(t)$ denote the theoretical survival function related with cause of death number i (i=1, ..., k). It is easy to show that in the frame of the PDRM model the following relations are true:

$$\frac{\mu_i(t)}{\mu_j(t)} = \frac{d\hat{S}_i(t)}{d\hat{S}_j(t)} \qquad (i,j = 1, ..., k) \tag{2}$$

where $\mu_i(t)$ is net mortality rate due to cause of death number i.

The relation (2) gives the proportion between the survival in the *contaminated population* and the mortality rates in the *pure population*. It may be used for estimation of the net mortality rates if any single rate is known from special medical studies. Suppose the net mortality rate due to cause of death number 1 is known. Then we may express the survival probability for cause of death number 1 in the form

$$\hat{S}_1(x) = 1 - \int_0^x \mu_1(t) \int \beta \, e^{-\beta \int_0^t \mu_1(\tau) \sum_{i=1}^{k} \frac{d\hat{S}_i(\tau)}{d\hat{S}_1(\tau)} d\tau} dP(\beta)\, dt \,. \tag{3}$$

The expression (3) is the integral equation of the Volterra kind with respect to the unknown distribution function $P(\beta)$. The equation (3) includes (k-1) unknown functions $\frac{d\hat{S}_i(\tau)}{d\hat{S}_1(\tau)}$ (i = 2, k). These functions may be estimated on the basis of the *contaminated population* cause-specific survival data. They are determined by the set of k integral equations

$$\hat{S}_1(t) = \int_0^t f(\tau)\, d\tau \tag{4}$$

$$\hat{S}_i(t) = \int_0^t \frac{d\hat{S}_i(\tau)}{d\hat{S}_1(\tau)} f(\tau)\, d\tau \qquad (i = 2, \ldots, k)\,. \tag{4}$$

Equations (3) may be solved after substituting the solution of set (4) into it.

The solution of the set (4) can be obtained by numeric statistical methods using the approach described in [2, 3]. The solution of equation (3) can be obtained by numeric statistical methods using the approach described in [2].

We may now write the expression for the cause-elimination survival function $\hat{S}_{\bullet r}(t)$ in a *contaminated population*. The formula uses solutions of equations (3) and (4) and may be expressed in the form

$$\hat{S}_{\bullet r}(t) = e^{-\int_0^t \varphi(\tau)\, K(\varphi(\tau))\, d\tau}$$

where

$$\varphi(\tau) = \mu_1(\tau) \sum_{i=1, i\neq r}^{k} \frac{d\hat{S}_i(\tau)}{d\hat{S}_1(\tau)}$$

$$K(a) = \frac{\int \beta\, e^{-a\beta}\, dP(\beta)}{\int e^{-a\beta}\, dP(\beta)}$$

$P(\beta)$ is the solution of equation (3) and

$\frac{dS_i(\tau)}{dS_1(\tau)}$ $(i = 2, \ldots, k)$ are solutions of (4).

Conclusions

The approach described in this paper should be considered as a step to understanding complex survival processes. The assumptions of the PDRM model are natural and the model may be considered as a step from a simple model of independent competing risks to a more sophisticated one.

The approach leads to integral equations of the Volterra kind with unstable solutions. Such equations need special numeric methods designed to assure solution stabilization. Some of these methods may be found in [2, 3].

References

1. Yashin AI, Manton KG, Vaupel JW (1985) Mortality and aging in heterogeneous population: a stochastic process model with observed and unobserved variables. Theor Pop Biol 27 (2):154-175
2. Michalski AI, Yashin AI (1986) Structural minimization of risk in estimation heterogeneity distributions. IIASA, Laxenburg, UP-86-76, p 25
3. Michalski AI (1987) Choice of an evaluation algorithm using samples of limited size. Automat Remote Control 36 (7):57-66

The Concept of Generalized Risk and Some Results of Preliminary Analysis

R. Prokhorskas

The effective use of health status models in planning disease prevention or health promotion programmes is rather exceptional. Ideally, an in-depth analysis, using appropriate models to simulate and test various prevention scenarios, should be an essential part of the planning process. In reality, the utilization of available epidemiological data is often limited only to inferring the existence of an association between risk factors and disease.

There is a variety of models of different complexity, designed to simulate the interaction between risk factors and morbidity or mortality. Unfortunately, in most cases they are still the subject of an academic interest of the scientific community, but not the real planning tool which might have a place on the desks of decision-makers at the Ministries of Health or other health authorities.

Potential users usually perceive health status models as interesting computer games and not as real planning tools. Different reasons could be listed for this distrust. Probably the most important is that the models are usually based on too many unverified assumptions or on data which are not accurate enough or convincing from the user's point of view. Most designers would admit that the main problems and weaknesses of their models are caused by the lack of data to estimate the parameters of a model. Very often a model is designed in such detail to simulate the disease process, that it is too complex to find sufficient data to *feed* into the model.

On the other hand, numerous prospective epidemiological studies over recent decades have generated a large amount of raw data on the association between risk factors and the risk of disease occurrence or of death. This is true, at least for some now commonly recognized risk factors such as smoking, high blood pressure and serum cholesterol. The problem is that the data are dispersed in small portions among the studies which have generated them. These data are not available or easily accessible to each model designer. An obvious solution is to pool these data, generalize the findings, and submit them in a ready-to-use form.

The Concept of Generalized Relative Risks

Only data requirements for health status models which are designed to simulate the changes of mortality in population in response to the changes in risk factors, are considered in this paper. With some simplifications, such models can be represented by a mathematical equation where the modifiable variable is the risk factor level, and the outcome variable is the mortality level. The analytical form of the equation reflects the existing knowledge on the association between risk factor(s) and health outcome.

To build such a model, at least two different types of data are needed. First, the distribution of risk factor(s) in the population under study. This data, if not readily available, can be obtained relatively easily by means of cross-sectional examination. The quantitative description of the association between risk factors and risk of death is the second type of data necessary to build the model. Large and expensive prospective studies, lasting at least five to ten years, are needed to produce this data. As mentioned above, a number of such studies have already been completed in several countries. Many of these demonstrate similar findings but each single study is too small to describe the risk factor and disease occurrence relationship in detail with a high level of statistical significance, and to provide evidence that the estimated associations are also valid in other populations. On the other hand, there is no reason to expect that the underlying risk association is different in different populations. On the contrary, the assumption of the common underlying risk association (at least for selected risk factors and health outcomes) is more realistic in epidemiologically similar populations. Otherwise, significant biological differences between populations resulting in difficult mechanisms of disease development would have to be accepted. Observable variations of the estimated risk association in different epidemiological studies can be explained by insufficient sample sizes, differences in methodology and usually unknown confounding factors. The amalgamation of relative risk estimates from as many studies as possible may result in developing generalized risk functions which could be considered as a *standard* association and would be more convincing for use in different countries and population groups, where no data are available to estimate the risk association.

It is obvious that the estimation of such generalized risk functions requires substantial efforts in order to collect data in a comparable form from a large number of studies.

The meta-analysis of published data cannot solve this problem as the data from single studies are usually analyzed and published in non-comparable or too aggregated forms.

A generalization is more simple and feasible at the level of relative risk than for the absolute risk, by assuming the multiplicative nature of the relationship between risk factor and mortality. The absolute risk (factor-specific mortality rate) could then be calculated, using the following transformation:

$$R(f=i) = \frac{R}{P(f=i) + (1-P(f=i))\ RR(f=i)^{-1}}$$

where

R(f=i)	absolute risk corresponding to the risk factor level i;
R	overall mortality for a given population (national mortality data is widely available);
P(f=i)	proportion of the population having a risk factor at level i;
RR(f=i)	generalized relative risk for risk factor at level i; i.e. risk ratio: risk factor equal to i/risk factor not equal to i.

The above formula can be used as a simple mortality model.

Preliminary Estimates of Generalized Risk

Analyses have been performed at the WHO Regional Office for Europe to obtain an impression of the applicability of a simple analytic scheme which will integrate risk estimates from different studies. The aim was to find average relative risk functions which describe the association between levels of blood pressure, serum cholesterol (CHOL), body mass index (BMI) and smoking with the risk of death from all causes, coronary heart disease (CHD) and cancer. The analyses were based on the assumption that the relative risks observed in the individual studies are randomly distorted measurements of a continuous underlying relative risk function. This hypothetical function was approximated by quadratic equation, assuming that the curve should be U-shaped, at least with regard to mortality from all causes. One can find a substantial number of studies confirming this expectation for biological risk factors such as body mass index or serum cholesterol. Regarding smoking, the risk ratio for smokers/nonsmokers was estimated.

The data used are limited to three prospective studies. They were originally designed to study cardiovascular diseases among middle-aged males. The main characteristics of the data are presented in Table 1.

Continuous risk factors were categorized in decile classes and the relative risk was then calculated for each class and study separately. The weighted averages were calculated in order to compare them with the quadratic approximation (Figures 1, 2, 3). The same analysis was repeated for different age-groups (40-45 and 50-60) and for age-adjusted factors for all ages. Age-

Table 1. Main characteristics of data used

Study	Age	*n*	Deaths Total	CHD	Cancer	Follow-up (years)
K1	44-60	2 455	480	96	117	11.8
RO	43-60	3 365	350	125	113	8.5
K2	38-61	5 679	329	91	81	6.9
Total	38-61	11 499	1 159	312	311	8.4

K1 = Kaunas part of WHO-Kaunas-Rotterdam Study - started in 1972
RO = Rotterdam part of above study
K2 = Multifactorial Coronary Heart Disease Prevention Study in Kaunas

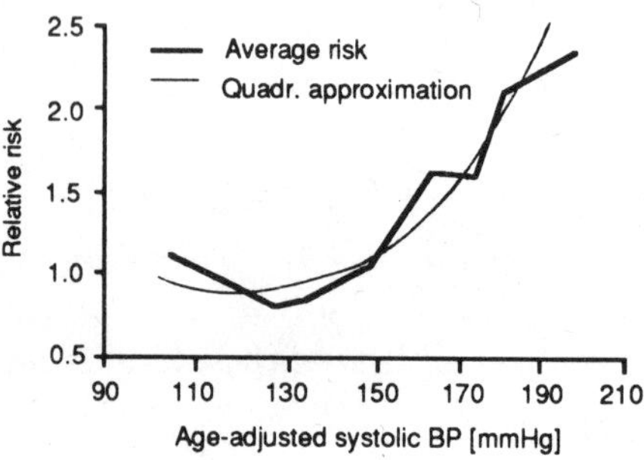

Fig. 1. Relative risk of total mortality in relation to systolic blood pressure

adjustment was made using a linear regression model with the age as the independent variable. The age-adjusted value of each risk factor was calculated as a mean value for the study plus a residual value.

Estimates of relative risk function for systolic and diastolic blood pressure (SBP, DBP), serum cholesterol and body mass index are given in Tables 2 and 3. The quadratic term for total mortality risk curve is significantly positive for all the above factors in the older age-group and for the age-adjusted values. The lower level of significance in the younger age-group might be explained by a smaller number of deaths occurring in this age-group. The minimum risk point for blood pressure is below the population average (respectively 124 and 137 mmHg for SBP; 80 and 85 mmHg for DBP). The risk is lowest at

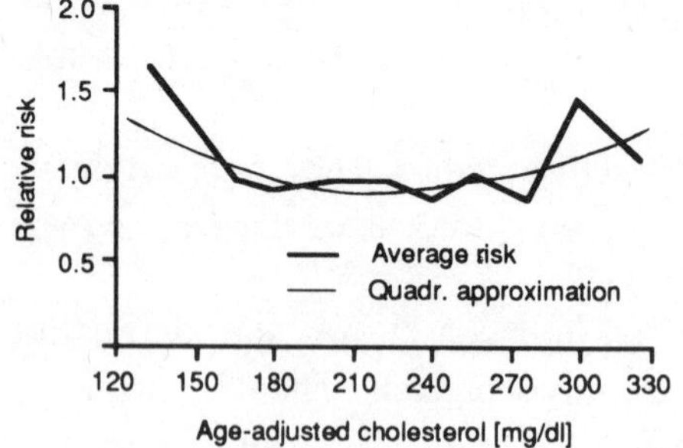

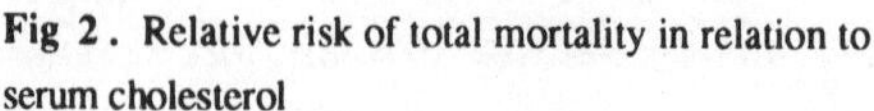

Fig 2. Relative risk of total mortality in relation to serum cholesterol

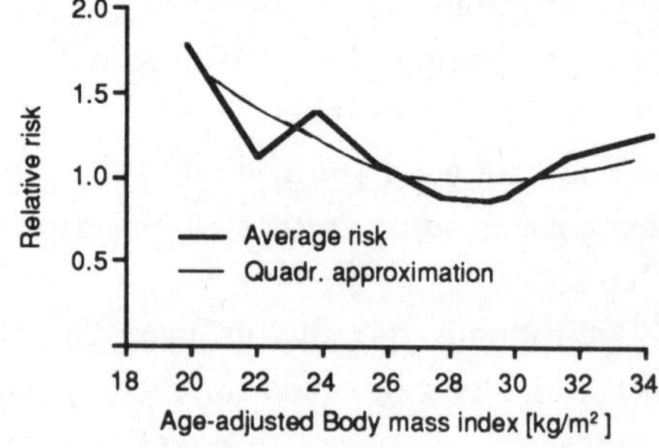

Fig. 3. Relative risk of total mortality in relation to serum cholesterol

Table 2. Parameters of quadratic approximation of total mortality relative risk

Risk factor	Age 40-49 Minimum risk point	Quadratic coefficient	p for quadratic coefficient	Age 50-60 Minimum risk point	Quadratic coefficient	p for quadratic coefficient
SBP	123.8	0.00058	0.001	125.0	0.00030	0.0002
DBP	79.4	0.00117	0.17	79.8	0.00091	0.0003
CHOL	215.4	0.000026	0.28	234.0	0.000062	0.008
BMI	29.3	0.00686	0.07	28.0	0.0126	0.0000

Table 3. Parameters of the quadratic approximation of relative risk function using age-adjusted factors

Risk factor	Total mortality Minimum risk point	Quadratic coefficient	p for quadratic coefficient	CHD mortality Minimum risk point	Quadratic coefficient	p for quadratic coefficient
SBP	124	0.00032	0.0001	92	0.00023	0.09
DBP	80.4	0.0011	0.0000	76.5	0.0012	0.0001
CHOL	232	0.000036	0.01	-1145	0.000003	0.9
BMI	28.5	0.0103	0.0000	27.2	0.0112	0.01
	Cancer mortality					
SBP	149	0.00009	0.3			
DBP	24	-0.00006	0.8			
CHOL	266	0.000055	0.06			
BMI	30.5	0.0095	0.001			

BMI level, about 28 kg/m^2, i.e. higher than the BMI average (27 kg/m^2). The minimum risk point for cholesterol is close to the average (233 mg/dl).

Estimates of the risk functions for CHD and cancer have markedly different parameters. The relationship of serum cholesterol and CHD mortality is practically linear. The large negative minimum risk value (-1145) is a consequence of this linear relationship.

It should be pointed out that the above estimates are illustrative, as they are based on data from only three studies. Data from more studies are needed to find risk estimates which would be applicable in practice.

Resource Allocation Models and Health Service Systems: an Exploration

A. R. Taket

Introduction

This paper reviews the subject of health services resource allocation models, and discusses some of the key factors in the choice of appropriate methods in order to develop an agenda for future work. It is divided into three main sections. The first considers different types of resource allocation problems encountered in health services, and identifies a classification of *problem areas*; it concludes by indicating which of these have been explored in theory and which in practice, in terms of application to real-world health systems. The second section analyzes factors affecting the choice of appropriate modelling approaches for particular problem areas. The third section presents four examples, relating to particular problem areas and resource allocation modelling approaches, and examines these in order to explore useful avenues for further development.

Problem Areas for Resource Allocation Models

The categorization of different areas of application for resource allocation models in the health services context is by no means simple. In this section, several different aspects of a situation in which such models might be applied are considered in turn, leading to the identification of different *problem areas*. The different aspects or factors that are considered, and the combinations which identify distinct problem areas, are summarized in Table 1 and are discussed below.

The first aspect to be considered is whether the area to be dealt with by the model is one of strategic or tactical planning. In many ways this simple strategic/tactical dichotomy represents an over-simplification of what is, in fact, a continuum in terms of the time period over which the resource allocation model is used. Strategic planning contexts typically are those where the time-scale considered is five years or longer, whereas tactical models may be concerned with the allocation of resources over the next year, month, week, or even day [1]. The task of strategic applications is essentially that of planning,

Table 1. Problem areas for resource allocation models

strategic or tactical application
level of application
national
regional
district
institution
nature of allocation required
geographical / spatial
patient type
treatment type
resource type
time periods
(and combinations)

whereas tactical applications are more concerned with management.

As earlier reviews have shown [2, 3], many resource allocation models of health service sectors or subsystems are intended for use in a highly localized tactical or operational planning context. Strategic planning is typically carried out at a fairly aggregate level in the health system; it is concerned largely with national or regional applications, rather than with the system defined by a single care unit (primary health care facility, clinic, hospital department, etc.) At the local district level, applications of both a strategic and tactical nature can be found.

The number and type of resources considered in the model are important. In some cases a single resource may be considered, and often requirements for resources of other types are estimated in proportion to this. Other models deal explicitly with several types of resource. A further distinction is made depending on whether costs are considered explicitly within the model; relatively few models exist where costs are completely specified. In terms of actual applications, hospital beds and various types of health manpower have been the types of resources most considered. This paper does not cover in detail the subject of resource allocation as applied to health manpower; an overview of approaches and a selected bibliography have been made by Thuriaux et al. [4].

The nature of the allocation required is also extremely important. Sometimes the issue is one of allocation of resources between different parts of the health system in a defined geographical area, for example between hospital and community care, where the question is one of allocating resources between different patient types. Other applications might be concerned with determining a suitable mix of different types of resources (for example staff, beds, and theatre time in a hospital) for one or more patient types, such applications being usually found at the tactical level. A slightly different problem is posed when the main question is the allocation of patients between different treatment types or *care packages*. Another question tackled is the time-scheduling of investment decisions concerning the opening of new or expanded facilities, or the closing of old facilities; this can be regarded as a problem of resource allocation between different time periods.

A different sort of resource allocation problem is the allocation of resources between different locations or geographical areas. Such applications may focus on a single type of resource, or may deal with questions of mixes of resources, different patient types, and/or different care packages. These more complex models are fewer in terms of actual applications, and are usually found at the tactical level. In any case, an important issue is how (or indeed whether) issues of accessibility to the population being served are incorporated into the model; existing applications deal with this issue with varying degrees of sophistication.

The classification of problem areas for resource allocation models, presented above, indicates a wide variety of situations where questions of resource allocation can arise. While most of these have been tackled in theoretical terms, practical applications have been more limited.

The Choice of Modelling Methodology

In this section, we review several factors that need to be taken into account in choosing an appropriate modelling methodology. These are summarized in Table 2, and are considered in turn.

Simulation versus Optimization and the Nature of Objectives

The distinction between modelling approaches based on optimization, and those based on simulation, is extremely important. An optimization approach is one which uses a model where the output is a single *optimum* or *best* allocation of resources, calculated to maximize (or minimize) an objective function. The use of such an approach is essentially *prescriptive*, in that the model generates a single *solution* to the resource allocation problem. However, there are often major difficulties in formulating a suitable objective function which incorporates all relevant criteria. For this reason, while the theoretical treatment of such optimization models is well developed, practical applications

Table 2. Issues in the choice of modelling methodology

simulation versus optimization and the nature of objectives
systemic constraints
the problem context
interaction between modeller and user(s)

remain rare. It is possible to use optimization models to generate different solutions or options in an iterative fashion, where the constraints in the model and/or the objective function for optimization are varied from iteration to iteration. The different solutions generated can then be judged in the light of criteria not explicitly incorporated in the model.

The simulation approach, on the other hand, is one where emphasis is on the use of models as decision-making aids in a resource allocation process, in order to explore the consequences of a series of possible resource allocation decisions in terms of one or more criteria/objectives of interest. The use of such models is *investigative* rather than prescriptive, and there is no direct generation of a *policy solution*. The models enable the consequences of different policy options to be explored in order to answer the question: *What happens if...?*, rather than attempting to produce an *optimum* solution. They require explicit generation, outside the model itself, of the range of policy options to be explored.

In most applications to date, the objectives used in resource allocation models have been fairly simple in nature, usually including only a single variable. Although modelling techniques exist which can deal with multiple objectives, real-world applications of these in the health service context are few and far between. As modelling techniques advance on the theoretical level, however, and also in terms of practicability owing to the increased availability of powerful computing facilities, this is an area that may well merit further development. This point is discussed further in later sections of this paper.

Sometimes, the objectives involve terms encompassing subjective value judgements (for example, about preferences for different treatment modalities or locations). These are sometimes obtained explicitly, and sometimes inferred or derived in the process of model calibration. There is a danger of modelling such judgements as if there were universal agreement on a single set of values (particularly in optimizing models). Models which attempt to incorporate different sets of values remain to be fully explored. This point is taken up later, when multiple criteria decision analysis (MCDA) is discussed.

Systemic Constraints on Resource Allocation

The types of problem areas identified in the first section were based on a focussed examination of the situation for which resource allocation decisions are required. To make an appropriate choice of methods, it is also necessary to examine the situation in a wider context, and this provides additional constraints on decision-making. Several issues are important here.

One issue is the need to recognize constraints that may be imposed by organizational and financial mechanisms controlling the health service system: market mechanisms if they exist, the nature and degree of any central control, and the limits on the freedom of the individual consumer/patient. These will determine whether the task of the model user is to respond to the actions of autonomous agents, or to initiate and direct usage. This brings us to the importance of users of the model, in terms of their roles and the degrees of freedom of action/decision available to them.

One must address the effects of all relevant and significant interactions in the health care system which may affect its behaviour, even if they are not explicitly the subject of the problem area concerned. An example of this is the interaction between the supply of, and demand for, different resources. It is widely accepted that, in many cases, the availability of a health care resource, in terms of its level and spatial distribution, will influence the demand for that resource. This, in turn, will affect the decisions made by health care professionals in allocating resources to patients and, ultimately, the level of use by different groups in the population. Many of the simpler resource allocation models ignore this interaction. Spatial interaction models have been used to simulate the resource allocation behaviour of various parts of the health care system, in order to provide tools for forecasting the consequences of future changes in population characteristics or resource availability, as an aid in allocating resources in the system. Some such models focus exclusively on locational issues, while others also incorporate other issues.

The Nature of the Problem Context

The third important issue in the choice of modelling methodology is the nature of the problem context in terms of the systems involved, the different participants/groups having an interest in the particular resource allocation problem, and the nature of their interactions. Building on the categorizations proposed by Jackson and Keys [5] and further developed by Jackson [6], a classification into six different types can be made, according to two factors:

- the nature of the systems involved in the problem area (either simple/mechanical or complex/systemic);
- the nature of the decision-makers or participants involved, and their interactions (unitary, pluralist, or coercive).

In terms of the first factor, the distinction is between systems consisting of a small number of elements whose interactions are observable, regular, and well-understood, and those characterized by a large number of elements which are highly interrelated, may be partially unobservable, and are affected by *behavioural* factors (political, cultural, ethical, etc.). Information on the problem area (as identified in terms of the aspects considered in the first section of this paper) allows us to categorize the nature of the systems involved. Within the health services setting, many tactical applications can be identified as simple/mechanical, while most strategic applications are complex/systemic.

In terms of the second factor in this classification (the nature of the participants involved and their interactions), unitary contexts are those where there is agreement between all decision-makers or participants on a common set of goals. In contrast, pluralist and coercive contexts are those where there is no such agreement. The distinction between pluralist and coercive contexts is made in terms of whether it is possible to bring about genuine compromise among the parties involved through negotiation (pluralist), or whether any *consensus* will be achieved through the exercise of power and domination, in which case the context is referred to as coercive. Such categorization may be made by examining the nature of the problem area and the systemic constraints on resource allocation, as discussed above. In terms of methods for resource allocation modelling, while there is a relative abundance of methods for unitary contexts and many examples of their successful application, there are fewer methods which are appropriate for pluralist contexts (some are discussed later), and fewer applications. Finally, it is uncertain whether appropriate methods exist for coercive contexts.

The problem context can also be categorized according to a third factor: the level of technical complexity that is appropriate for use. The concept of *appropriateness* can be applied in at least two different ways. The first relates to the level of specialist help available, in terms of skilled personnel, computing facilities, and other resources. The second interpretation relates to the level of complexity with which the users of the model (i.e. the decision-makers/participants) feel at ease. It is debatable which of these interpretations should be dominant, but the wider the gap between the two in any particular situation, the harder it will be to achieve successful implementation and continued use of the resource allocation model.

Degree of Interaction between Modeller and User

Finally, the choice of methodology will be influenced by the degree of interaction that is possible between the modeller and the decision-maker. This will lie within a range from no direct involvement at all to a fully interactive collaboration in developing and using the model concerned. Lack of any direct involvement will severely limit the options in terms of methodology; for example, where value judgements are to be incorporated, they will have to be inferred. When higher levels of interaction are possible, an increased range of methods becomes available.

This factor will affect not only the choice of method, but also the likelihood of successful implementation. It is also closely related to (but conceptually distinct from) the level of technical complexity that is appropriate for use (discussed earlier). It is thus important that these two aspects should be considered together.

Developing Models for the Future: Towards an Agenda for Action

This final section presents four specific examples, drawing on the preceding discussion, to illustrate a range of areas where work can usefully be developed. Table 3 illustrates how they fit into the schema discussed in the first two sections of the paper.

Equity and Accessibility as Objectives: Spatial Interaction Modelling and the Allocation of Resources across Space

Spatial interaction modelling, or gravity modelling, provides a means of representing aggregate service utilization patterns in terms of three broad groups of factors that are known to influence the uptake of services: the level and type of facilities provided at different locations; the relative need for services in communities in different localities, i.e. the community morbidity; and the physical accessibility of the facilities to the different communities. It is not assumed that patients visit their nearest facility, or that each community is assigned to the catchment area of a single facility, so the method can deal with the complex pattern of cross-boundary flows that exist in practice.

This type of modelling approach to health service systems was just applied in the USA [7, 8, 9]. In the late 1970's, work started in the UK to examine the patterns of flow of inpatients within the four Thames Regional Health Authorities [10], as a result of the London Health Planning Consortium study of acute hospital services in London [11]. The resulting models can be used to help explore the potential consequences for the populations living in the various parts of the region under study, of different strategic planning options under consideration for relocation of acute hospital facilities. In particular, they can be used to explore the likely effects of changes in the supply pattern of facilities

Table 3. Developing models for the future - towards an agenda for action

Examples	Problem area	Methodological approach
Equity and accessibility as objectives: spatial interaction modelling and the allocation of resources across space	• strategic • regional or below • geographical/spatial	• simulation • assumption of no change in referral mechanisms • pluralist, complex • some interaction
Efficiency as an objective: the use of data envelopment analysis	• strategic or tactical • district or institution • between resource types	• optimization • assumption of no change in underlying production functions • pluralist, complex • no interaction
The balance of care approach: resource allocation for a client group	• strategic or tactical • district or institution • between patient, treatment and resource type, across time	• simulation/ optimization • pluralist, simple • medium to high interaction
Multiple criteria decision analysis and resource allocation models	• strategic or tactical • district or institution • dependent on particular models used	• simulation • pluralist, simple or complex • high interaction

and/or population movement on measures of equity (use in relation to need) and access (travel time or distance to hospital) for different communities. The models are used to explore the consequences of options which have already been established as feasible, under other constraints on the expansion or contraction of facilities on existing sites, as well as the potential for development of new sites. The information provided by the models forms one of the inputs into the decision-making process associated with strategic planning.

Similar models are now in use in other European countries, as well as in Australia and the USA [12]. In the UK, several Regional Health Authorities (RHAs) have used a gravity model approach in strategic planning, for example the North-East Thames RHA [13], the West Midlands RHA [14], and the East Anglian RHA [15]. The mathematical formulations for typical models are shown in the Annex.

There are several potential areas for future work. First is the continued development of methodological and computational aspects of the analysis of equity and accessibility issues, in particular questions about the appropriate geographical scales for modelling, the nature of patient classification, and the specification of appropriate measures of accessibility. Secondly, in the context of an increased emphasis on the introduction of market mechanisms into health service systems in many European countries, the relevance of such modelling approaches needs to be re-assessed. Owing to the nature of the changes proposed in the ways services are organized and provided, considerable re-specification of the models may be necessary. Thirdly, it should be noted that, as yet, practical applications are found only for hospital-based services [12]. A major reason for this is that data are more readily available in the inpatient sector. This is likely to change, however, with the increasing use of IT in health service systems, and in particular in the primary health care sector, which should make it more feasible to investigate the application of spatial interaction modelling to all sectors of the health system. Fourthly, previous work in this field [15, 16] has shown the potential conflicts that can arise between objectives of equity and accessibility. In this area, it would be useful to extend the use of the models to explicit consideration of trade-offs between the two objectives. Detailed proposals for research in the UK to address these questions are under preparation.

So far, the measures of need used in these models have been rather simple, and based on the concept of comparative need in Bradshaw's taxonomy [17]. It would be valuable to investigate the use of outputs from health status models to refine the measures of need used; this would represent a shift towards measures based more on normative need. This is by no means a new idea, as linkages of this type were foreshadowed in the strategy adopted for work carried out or proposed at IIASA [18], and elsewhere [19, 20]. However, practical applications have not yet been widely implemented. The problems are due, at least in part, to differences in the patient types covered by health status models and spatial interaction models. Typically, the applications of spatial interaction models have focussed on the totality of inpatient admissions, or on broad specialty groups, sometimes subdivided into elective and non-elective admissions. Health status models, on the other hand, usually tackle single diagnostic categories, so that the outputs from several linked models would be required. Although the disaggregation of spatial interaction models by specialty presents no theoretical difficulties, the performance of such models has not given a sufficiently accurate replication of observed usage to be used for resource allocation. Evidence from such applications in the UK suggests that this is at least partially due to the problem of classifying patients into specialties (on the basis of the admitting consultant's designation, rather than on patient diagnosis), and to the indistinct and variable boundaries between inpatient admission, day care, and outpatient care. These problems, and other problems of data availability and accuracy, can be partially remedied by greater use of more sophisticated information systems throughout the health services, although recent investigations [21, 22] into patient and other information systems, in one district and one region in England, indicate that considerable problems still remain.

Efficiency as an Objective: the Use of Data Envelopment Analysis

Data envelopment analysis (DEA) is a relatively novel approach to the measurement of relative efficiency across a number of units, where there are multiple incommensurate inputs and outputs. In the health service context, the units might be hospitals, other types of health care facility, or geographical districts. The application of DEA for use in resource allocation comes from its ability to identify sets of peer units, and to set targets for inefficient units by reference to the performance characteristics of other peer units. Such targets can then be used in the allocation of resources. The approach originated in papers by Farrell [23] and Farrell and Fieldhouse [24], while the target-setting applications of DEA are discussed by Thanassoulis and Dyson [25]. The mathematical formulation is shown in the Annex.

The advantage of the DEA approach is its recognition that it is legitimate for different units (hospitals, health authorities, etc.) to value inputs and outputs differently in any assessment of efficiency. In comparing units, DEA seeks to find, for each unit in turn, the valuation of inputs and outputs that shows the unit in the most favourable light in comparison to all other units in the set.

So far, this technique has seldom been applied in the health systems setting. Some preliminary investigators in England and Wales, using districts and hospitals as the units for analysis, have focussed on the use of DEA for assessing performance and efficiency, but have not yet been developed into resource allocation applications. The range of outputs has also been rather limited. As information availability improves, the method may merit further examination. But it is not without potential problems, in particular:

- the difficulty of including all relevant inputs and outputs;
- the aggregate level at which such analysis operates, to avoid including too many input and output variables in relation to the number of units;
- the implicit assumptions made about economies of scale (although more sophisticated assumptions can be incorporated);
- units with particularly unusual patterns of inputs and outputs may appear efficient. This may not reflect *real* efficiency, but rather a sparse or empty set of peer units. Ways round this problem might involve imposing further restrictions on the weights applied to different inputs and outputs, but there is then the problem of justifying the nature and extent of such restrictions;
- whether environmental factors (such as social deprivation) can be adequately represented in the formulation.

So although the potential of this approach remains to be fully explored, this paper should not be interpreted as making an unqualified assertion that it will prove a suitable technique for widespread use. Given the points raised above, its major applications may be found in the tactical arena, and for specific, well-defined patient categories.

The Balance of Care Approach: Resource Allocation for a Client Group

The balance of care (BOC) model has by now a long and somewhat checkered history, during which the nature of the modelling approaches adopted has changed radically. This history is of considerable relevance in identifying general barriers to widespread use of resource allocation modelling, and so will be reviewed briefly here.

The BOC model had its origins in modelling work developed by the Department of Health and Social Security (DHSS) in the UK [26], which examined the allocation of resources for health and personal social services. The model used the current amounts of resources allocated to different categories of patients to infer the value judgements of professional workers in the field. These were then used to estimate (by a technique of non-linear mathematical programming) how the field workers would allocate any given mix of resources that might be provided (a simulation type of approach), and what would be the *best* set of resources to be provided (an optimization type of approach), where the inferred value judgements of the field workers were used to define *best*. The model took into account the limitation of resources, the competition for resources between services or care groups, the interrelationships between services, and the availability of alternative forms of care.

The BOC model was used in different regions of the UK [27, 28], as well as in a national planning context [29], and in some other regions, for example Western Australia [30]. A closely related model, DRAM (disaggregated resource allocation model), was later developed at the IIASA as one of a family of health systems models. DRAM's formulation, history, and use have been outlined by Hughes and Taket [31].

Despite considerable theoretical development, and some practical applications, use of the original BOC or of DRAM remains rare. In addition to technical criticisms, which in the case of the BOC model focussed particularly on the derivation and use of *inferred worth*, the models were seen as rather opaque and *unfriendly* by their potential users. The computational requirements, the data requirements, the level of involvement of health personnel in the calibration stages, and the technical expertise required to *interpret* the model's output to the planner or decision-maker all contributed to their lack of use.

For this reason, a revised version of the BOC model was developed [32], using less complex modelling techniques, and designed to be simpler for planners to understand and use. It has been used at district level in the UK [33]. The simplification and clarification of the model did not, however, go so far as to guarantee its widespread use, and this has resulted in yet further versions of the BOC model, this time specifically for elderly people. The first version [34] uses currently available data to generate estimates of the numbers of elderly people with particular types of care needs, and allows users to explore the resource implications of a range of care options. It uses a proprietary spreadsheet package for use on a micro-computer. The system consists of two parts: a population model and a care options model. The former provides estimates of the numbers of elderly people in a given locality, in each of a number of dependency categories. In the care options model, the resource implications of the population model are explored, initial sets of care options are provided for each dependency category (these can be adjusted as required by the user), and the resource allocation can be made on the basis of minimum cost, specified preference, or the allocation that was observed in some locality (usually obtained through a special survey). The consequences of the allocation, in terms of service levels and costs, are presented to the user. The user is then allowed to go back and readjust care options and/or allocation criteria, and to examine the resultant differences in allocations, service levels, and costs.

This system was released in 1987, and was acquired by over half of the 200 or so health authorities in England and Wales [35]. Precise details of the extent and depth of use are hard to come by, but feedback to the DHSS has resulted in yet further re-specification and re-packaging of the system [36]. These latest modifications include changes to the user interface, and changes to the specification of dependency categories based on a recent national disability survey. In all these later versions of the model, the dependency categories used are derived from single cross-sectional surveys or combinations thereof. A similar modelling approach has also been applied to the planning of services related to HIV and AIDS [37, 38]. Further development is planned for other client groups, for example the physically disabled and the mentally ill.

These later versions of the BOC model offer several possibilities for the use of outputs from health status modelling. One would be in the population model, to refine the dependency categories used, and also to include the time dimension explicitly, through use of outputs concerning life expectancy in different dependency categories. This sort of development and refinement of the population model component would give the BOC model improved potential for use in a strategic time framework. Outputs from health status models could also be used in the care options model, to help delineate appropriate packages of care.

Looking at the history of the BOC model, two developments can be observed. The first is one of progressive mathematical simplification: away from optimization, inferred worth, and mathematical programming towards simulation using much simpler input/output equations. The second is changes in the nature of the interaction between modeller and user, from an almost complete separation of the two, through various intermediate stages, to the latest version where the user to some extent becomes the modeller, through being able to specify and adjust model inputs, such as care options. Experience using the latest version of the model suggests that technical mediation or facilitation is still required, and it remains to be seen whether this will still be so once the latest modifications are completed. Extensive testing in this area is planned.

It was noted above that the outputs from the model are presented to the user in terms of both service levels and costs. Recent developments in MCDA (discussed below) may provide improved ways of presenting such information to the user so as to facilitate choices between different resource configurations.

Finally, in terms of trends in the development of the model, we have noticed an increased emphasis, in later versions, on the process by which resource allocation decisions are considered by the relevant parties. This, again, is an area where developments in MCDA, and in so-called *soft* OR approaches, have much potential that remains to be fully explored.

Multiple Criteria Decision Analysis (MCDA) and Resource Allocation Models

The basis of MCDA approaches is the desire to take account of multiple, and possibly conflicting, criteria in a decision-making process. The use of MCDA in resource allocation modelling arose from a recognition that the *application* of resource allocation models to real-world health systems involves what is essentially a decision-making process.

A recent review of methodology in the area of MCDA [39] usefully summarizes five key points which underlie its potential for use (my *italics* in the following quoting):

- 'multiple criteria approaches seek to take *explicit* account of multiple conflicting criteria in aiding decision-making;
- the principal aim is to help decision-makers *learn* about their own and others' values and judgements, and through organization, synthesis and appropriate presentation of information to *guide them* in identifying, often through intensive discussion, a preferred course of action;
- the most useful approaches are conceptually *simple and transparent*;
- *there is a skill in making effective use of a simple tool* in a potentially complex environment;
- the process leads to *better considered*, justifiable and explainable decisions.'

It is also useful to distinguish between two types of circumstance in which MCDA may be used [40, 41]:

- to evaluate and choose between a number of discretely defined alternatives (sometimes referred to as multi-attribute decision-making), in the resource allocation context, between a number of pre-determined possible allocations of resources;
- to identify a preferred alternative from a potentially infinite set of alternatives implicitly defined by a set of constraints (sometimes referred to as multiple-objective decision-making), in the resource allocation context, to identify a preferred allocation of resources. Note that this is not strictly equivalent to an optimization type of approach, since there is no requirement to identify only one preferred option.

Belton [39] distinguishes these two types as the evaluation problem and the design problem, respectively.

Applications of MCDA in the health field are as yet rare. A recent review [42] of applications which used multiple objective methods, and were published between 1955 and 1986, classifies applications in terms of status with regard to implementation and methods used. Of the 504 references classified, 58 had been implemented; of the 13 which describe applications in the health services field, only one was classified as having been implemented in practice.

Some potential areas for development of MCDA are as follows: one is the application of computer-based, visual interactive approaches to goal programming, which allows the user/decision-maker to explore sets of feasible resource allocation options interactively, while monitoring their effect on objectives of interest, developing, for example, along the lines of Kohonen and Laasko [43]. A potential application of this, in the context of extensions of the BOC approach discussed earlier and the challenge to development in this direction, would be to maintain sufficient transparency to the user. A second possible area for development is the use of methods developed through work on the *evaluation problem* within MCDA. Here, an interesting application could be to the use of outputs from spatial interaction models (discussed earlier) relating to different criteria, such as equity and access. Similar applications could be to the use of outputs from other models. In both cases, the potential benefits are linked to the use of increased computer power, and the adoption of an essentially interactive approach to the problem of resource allocation modelling.

Conclusions

In conclusion, some of the issues raised above can be highlighted. The nature of such *conclusions* remains provisional and tentative however, until the developments in methods, and the use of methods, discussed in the paper are carried out in practice.

Firstly, there remain a number of theoretical tools whose usefulness for health services resource allocation modelling remains to be explored. A general theme underlying many suggestions is one of increased interaction between the modeller and the user, and this is reflected in an increased emphasis on the process of implementation or application of resource allocation modelling, rather than on refinements to the technical specifications of the models used. This is not to suggest that such refinements are unnecessary (far from it!), and some avenues requiring development have already been identified in this paper. Rather, the intention is to suggest that decision-making processes involved in the use of resource allocation models are an extremely important part of the total picture.

A related issue is how to achieve sufficient involvement of the relevant parties in the project; this remains problematic, and is an area requiring further attention. We might also note that putting emphasis on interaction and the decision-making process has implications for the portability/transferability of resource allocation models.

Many of the suggestions for further development have become available only through continued developments in IT. Still further possibilities, not even touched on in this paper, might involve investigating the use of expert systems technologies in resource allocation.

Other underlying trends are a move towards explicit incorporation of subjective elements in the formulation and use of models, the adoption of a simulation rather than an optimization approach, and the recognition of multiple objectives and different value systems. This area could not be explored in detail in this paper. However, a whole range of techniques, the so-called *soft* OR approaches [44], have the potential for helping to elicit and structure subjective elements.

In many European countries, the rapidly changing nature of health systems, in terms of their financing, organization, and referral mechanisms, poses particular challenges to resource allocation modelling. The consequences of this are likely to include a need for models to be re-specified, re-calibrated, and validated before being transferred for use in a different setting to that of their origin. This is another factor hindering the easy portability of resource allocation models. A related problem is the difficulty of finding appropriate models for use in coercive contexts (where all relevant participants do not agree about a common set of goals, and where it is not possible to bring about genuine accommodation among the parties involved through negotiation), and even of defining what *appropriate* might mean in such contexts.

Annex

Spatial Interaction Models

Attraction constrained:

$$T_{ik} = B_k D_k W_i f(b, c_{ik})$$

where

i, k	index the origin and destination zones, respectively
T_{ik}	is the flow of patients from zone i to zone k for treatment
D_k	is the capacity of destination zone k to treat patients
W_i	is a measure of the relative need of residents in zone i (the patient generating factor for zone i)
$f(b, c_{ik})$	the deterrence function
b	a parameter determined during calibration
c_{ik}	a measure of the accessibility of hospitals in treatment zone k to residents of area i

B_k $= (\sum_i W_i f(b, c_{ik}))^{-1}$ (which ensures that $\sum_i T_{ik} = D_k$) .

Production constrained:

$$T_{ik} = B_i A_k W_i f(b, c_{ik})$$

where

i, k	index the origin and destination zones, respectively
T_{ik}	is the flow of patients from zone i to zone k for treatment
A_k	is the attractiveness of destination zone k
W_i	is the demand from residents in zone i
$f(b, c_{ik})$	the deterrence function
b	a parameter determined during calibration
c_{ik}	a measure of the accessibility of hospitals in treatment zone k to residents of area i
B_i	$= (\sum_k A_k f(b, c_{ik}))^{-1}$ (which ensures that $\sum_k T_{ik} = W_i$) .

Data Envelopment Analysis

Algebraically, the DEA problem can be formulated as follows:
Define a common measure of relative efficiency as the ratio of a weighted sum of outputs to a weighted sum of inputs, and let

x_{ij}	the amount of input i used by unit j
y_{kj}	the amount of output k produced by unit j
u_{ir}	the weight given to input i which produces the highest relative efficiency for unit r
v_{kr}	the weight given to output k which produces the highest relative efficiency for unit r

and

E_{jr}	the relative efficiency for unit j under the weights which produce the highest relative efficiency for unit r:

$$= \frac{\sum_k v_{kr}\, y_{kj}}{\sum_i u_{ir}\, x_{ij}} .$$

Then it is required to find u_{ir}, v_{kr} to maximise E_{jr} for each r in turn, subject to

$E_{jr} \leq 1$

$u_{ij} > e$

$v_{kj} > e$

where e is a small positive quantity.

This is equivalent to solving a single linear programming problem for each of the units in turn. Units where E_{rr} are strictly less than one represent those whose relative efficiency is not optimum, relative to the other units in the comparison set.

References

1. Jardel JP, Miltenyi K, Taket AR (1986) Interactive models and other systems approaches: a review of methods. In: Health projections in Europe - methods and applications. World Health Organization Regional Office for Europe, Copenhagen, pp 173-189
2. Clayden D, Boldy D (eds) (1977) Current operational research problems in health and welfare services in the United Kingdom and Ireland. Operational Research Society, Birmingham, p 53
3. Tunnicliffe-Wilson JC (1980) A review of operational problems tackled by computer simulation in health care facilities. Health and Social Services Journal 90:73-80
4. Thuriaux MC, Knight JE, Lopez AD (1986) Projections of health resources and their use: methods and data requirements. In: Health projections in Europe - methods and applications. World Health Organization Regional Office for Europe, Copenhagen, pp 93-104
5. Jackson MC, Keys P (1984) Towards a system of systems methodologies. Journal of the Operational Research Society 33:473-486
6. Jackson MC (1990) Beyond a system of systems methodologies. Journal of the Operational Research Society 41:657-668
7. Morrill RL, Kelley M (1970) The simulation of hospital use and the estimation of location efficiency. Geographical Analysis 2:283-299
8. Trebbi G (1972) Planning regional inpatient facilities. In: Proceedings of the Third Annual Pittsburgh Conference on Modelling and Simulation. Instrument Society of America, Pittsburgh
9. Ault D et al. (1974) The effects of suburban hospital construction on the occupancy rates of central city hospitals. In: Proceedings of the Fifth Annual Pittsburgh Conference on Modelling and Simulation. Instrument Society of America, Pittsburgh
10. Taket AR, Mayhew LD (1981) Interactions between the supply of and demand for hospital services in London. Omega 9 (5):519-526
11. London Health Planning Consortium (1979) Acute hospital services in London. HMSO, Department of Health and Social Security, London, p 72

12. Taket AR, Mayhew LD, Gibberd RW, Hall NM, Bevan RG, Wanng D, Bertuglia CS, Tadei R, Risung EJ (1986) RAMOS: a model of the spatial allocation of health care resources. In: Health projections in Europe - methods and applications. World Health Organization Regional Office for Europe, Copenhagen, pp 218-236
13. Stone J (1984) Predicting patient flows to local acute hospitals. In: van Eimeren W, Engelbrecht R, Flagle CD (eds) Proceedings of the third international conference on system science and health care. Springer, Berlin Heidelberg New York, pp 1013-1016
14. Clare PH, Churchill KE (1989) The application of gravity modelling to regional strategic planning with particular attention to forecasting catchments of new hospitals. West Midlands Regional Health Authority, Management Services Division, Birmingham, p 21
15. Taket AR (1989) Equity and access: exploring the effects of hospital location on the population served. Journal of the Operational Research Society 40 (11):1001-1009
16. Taket AR (1990) Measuring inequalities in health service provision. Paper presented at Regional European Meeting of the International Epidemiological Association, Granada, Spain, February 1990 (unpublished)
17. Bradshaw J (1972) The concept of social need. New Society (30 March 1972):640-643
18. Chigan EN, Hughes DJ, Kitont P (1979) Health care systems modelling at IIASA: a status report. IIASA, Laxenburg, SR-79-4, p 24
19. Clarke M, Forte P, Spowage M, Wilson AG (1984) A strategic planning simulation model of a district health service system, the inpatient component and results. In: van Eimeren W, Engelbrecht R, Flagle CD (eds) Proceedings of the third international conference on system science and health care. Springer, Berlin Heidelberg New York, pp 949-954
20. Lagergren M (1984) Future resource requirements for health care - a modelling approach. In: van Eimeren W, Engelbrecht R, Flagle CD (eds) Proceedings of the third international conference on system science and health care. Springer, Berlin Heidelberg New York, pp 938-941
21. Saleeb S (1989) Report of the mismatch study for the proposed community index. Department of Community Medicine, Tower Hamlets Health Authority, London, p 73
22. Taket AR (1990) Hospitalization for Tower Hamlets residents: a preliminary analysis. Paper presented at a day conference on research into hospitalization. Academic Centre, Newham General Hospital, North East Thames Regional Health Authority (unpublished)
23. Farrell MJ (1957) The measurement of productive efficiency. Journal of the Royal Statistical Society A 120:253-281
24. Farrell MJ, Fieldhouse M (1962) Estimating efficient production functions under increasing returns to scale. Journal of the Royal Statistical Society A 125:252-267
25. Thanassoulis E, Dyson RG (1988) Setting target input and output levels for relative efficiency under different priorities over individual input output improvements (Warwick Papers in Management No 25). University of Warwick, Warwick, p 37
26. McDonald AG, Cuddeford CG, Beale EJL Mathematical models of the balance of care. British Medical Bulletin:262-270

27. Canvin R, Hansan J, Lyons I, Russel JC (1972) Balance of care in Devon: joint strategic planning of health and social services at AHA and county level. Health and Social Services Journal 88:C17-C20
28. Boldy D, Canvin R, Russel I, Roystron G (1981) Planning the balance of care. In: Boldy D (ed) Operational research applied to the health services. Croom Helm, London, pp 84-108
29. Gibbs RJ (1978) The use of a strategic planning model for health and personal social services. Journal of the Operational Research Society 29 (9):875-883
30. Boldy DP, Rhys-Hearn C (1984) Strategies for assessing and monitoring appropriate long-term costs for elderly people. In: van Eimeren W, Engelbrecht R, Flagle CD (eds) Proceedings of the third international conference on system science and health care. Springer, Berlin Heidelberg New York, pp 199-202
31. Hughes DJ, Taket AR (1986) DRAM: a model of health care resource allocation. In: Health projections in Europe - methods and applications. World Health Organization Regional Office for Europe, Copenhagen, pp 191-218
32. Klemperer PD, McClenahan JW (1981) Joint strategic planning between health and local authorities. Omega:481-492
33. Borley RG et al. (1981) Balance of care - a user's view of a new approach to joint strategic planning. Omega 9 (5):493-500
34. Bowen T, Forte P (1987) The Balance of care microcomputer system: guidance for users. Operational Research Service, Department of Health and Social Security, London, p 24
35. Forte P, Bowen T (1988) A microcomputer system for planning the balance of care for elderly people. In: Duru G, Engelbrecht R, Flagle CD, van Eimeren W (eds) System Science in Health Care. Masson 3, Paris, pp 363-366
36. Lord J (1990) Community care planning and the balance of care system. Paper presented to the 32nd Conference of the Operational Research Society, Bangor, Wales, (unpublished)
37. Bowen T, Forte P, Smith M (1990) A service planning model for HIV and AIDS. In: Dangerfield BC Roberts CA (eds) OR work in HIV/AIDS. Operational Research Society, Birmingham, pp 23-25
38. Rosenhead JR, Reddington K, Rizakou K (1990) Planning for HIV and AIDS in a Health District. In: Dangerfield BG, Roberts CA (eds) OR work in HIV/AIDS. Operational Research Society, Birmingham, pp 27-31
39. Belton V (1990) Multiple criteria decision analysis - practically the only way to choose.In: Hendry LC, Eglese RW (eds) Operational research tutorial papers 1990. Operational Research Society, Birmingham, pp 53-101
40. Hwang CL, Masud ASM (1979) Multiple objective decision-making. Springer, Berlin Heidelberg New York
41. Hwang CL, Yoon K (1981) Multiple attribute decision-making. Springer, Berlin Heidelberg New York, p 259
42. White DJ (1990) A bibliography on the application of mathematical programming multiple-objective methods. Journal of the Operational Research Society 41 (8):669-691

43. Kohonen P, Laasko J (1986) A visual interactive method for solving the multiple criteria problem. European Journal of Operational Research 24:277-287
44. Rosenhead JR (ed) (1989) Rational analysis for a problematic world. Wiley, Chichester, p 370

Micro Simulation of Costs and Effects: the Case of Heart Transplantation

B. A. van Hout and J. D. F. Habbema

Introduction

Technology assessment is an important aid in monitoring the introduction of new medical procedures. These are evaluated from a medical, economic, social, ethical, and legal aspects so as to facilitate rational decision-making by the authorities. The Dutch heart transplant evaluation study is an example of this type of research, in which emphasis was placed on costs and effects. The study was initiated in 1985, one year after the first Dutch heart transplant. It served two goals. First, it aimed to reach consensus about the introduction of heart transplantation into the Dutch health care system. Second, it was one of several studies intended to explore the usefulness of cost-effectiveness health care.

In cost-effectiveness analysis, costs and effects of a defined health care programme are compared with costs and effects of alternatives. The most plausible alternative to heart transplantation is optimal conventional treatment without transplantation. Therefore, the costs and effects of a heart transplant programme have been compared with costs and effects without such a programme. For this purpose, separate analyses were conducted regarding survival [1], costs [2], and quality of life [3], all with and without a transplant programme. In addition, separate studies were carried out regarding the future number of donor hearts [4] and the number of future patients who were expected to be referred to the programme [5]. Results from all these studies were integrated in a model which was used to forecast the future development of the Dutch heart transplant programme [6].

In the model, different treatment stages (compartments) are defined, and durations within these stages are handled as stochastic variables. Thus the model may be labelled as a stochastic compartment model [7].

Micro-simulation was chosen as the appropriate technique for calculations. Using this technique, account can be taken of interactions between the number of patients on the waiting list, survival probabilities, the number of donor-organs, and matching criteria between donors and recipients [8]. The direct result of the micro-simulation technique consists of patient histories containing patient characteristics and precise data on entering and leaving the different treatment stages. Costs and effects are secondary results, obtained by adding up durations and by linking patient histories to estimates of costs and quality of life corresponding to the different treatment stages.

This paper presents the Dutch heart transplant model. It also shows that the structure of micro-simulation fits in perfectly with the results of survival analysis applied to the durations of subsequent compartments. As such, it is a powerful tool in calculating costs and effects in stochastic compartment models.

The Dutch Heart Transplant Programme

After the first Dutch heart transplant on 23 June 1984, Dutch health care authorities licensed two transplant centres to perform a limited number of heart transplants. The first centre is shared by three hospitals: the University Hospital in Rotterdam, the University Hospital in Leiden, and the St. Anthonius Hospital in Nieuwegein. The second centre is shared by two hospitals: the University Hospital in Utrecht and the University Hospital in Groningen. The operations were performed in only two hospitals, the University Hospitals in Rotterdam and Utrecht, where organization and administration were also centralized.

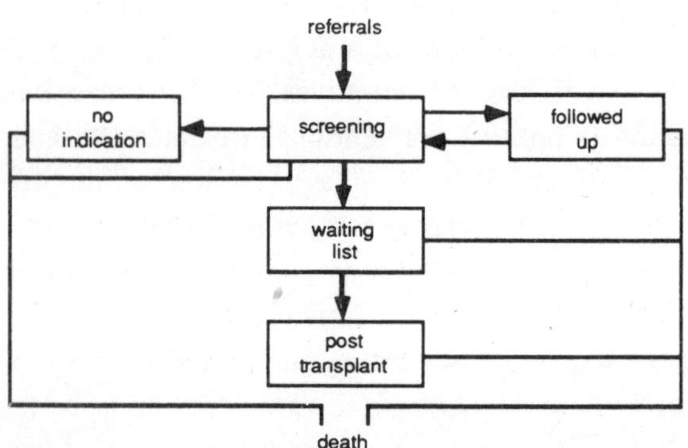

Fig. 1. The Dutch Heart Transplant Programme, flow chart model

The decision structure of the Dutch heart transplant programme is shown in Figure 1. After referral to a transplant centre, a patient is screened to determine if a transplant is indicated. After screening, three decisions are possible. First, a transplant is definitely not indicated, the patient returns to the referring hospital. Second, a transplant is not indicated but might be in the future (for example, if the patient's condition is not severe enough, or if some other treatment is still possible, which may be medical therapy or conventional càrdiac surgery), the patient returns to the referring hospital, but contact is retained with the transplant centre. Third, a transplant is indicated and the patient is placed on the waiting list; further treatment is carried out by the transplant centre. If a patient has no indication for heart transplant but might have in the future, he may return to the transplant centre to be screened for a second or even a third time. After referral to the waiting list, a patient is either transplanted or dies awaiting transplant. After transplantation, no further refinement in treatment stages is made.

From 1983 to 1988, 346 patients were referred to the two centres (238 to Amsterdam, 108 to Utrecht). Seventy-six transplants were performed (57 in Rotterdam and 19 in Utrecht). It was decided that a transplant was not indicated for 79 patients. Ninety-five patients were referred to the waiting list of Eurotransplant (an international organization which coordinates organ transplants). One patient was removed from this list, 75 were transplanted (one of them for a second time), and sixteen died waiting for a donor heart. Thirty-seven patients died before any formal decision about further treatment was made, and 15 died while they were registered in the *follow-up* group.

Both centres provided data on all patients who had been referred during the years 1984-87. The data included socio-demographic and medical characteristics, and flow-chart data. Data collection on costs was restricted to those periods when patients were treated in Rotterdam or Utrecht. Data on quality of life were obtained from computer-assisted interviews in 1986-87, according to a three-month schedule, from patients who had been transplanted or who had not yet been transplanted.

The Model

The Dutch heart transplant programme was modelled according to treatment stages, which were defined following the decision structure within the programme. Basically, the model distinguishes the following input sources:

- forecasts of the annual number of patients referred to the transplant centres;
- forecasts of the annual number of donor hearts;
- estimates of duration-distributions.

Secondary input sources are:

- estimates of costs;
- estimates of quality-of-life indicators.

Different values of input sources imply different scenarios. Two scenarios have been central to the analysis: the base-line scenario and the non-transplant scenario. In the base-line scenario, the consequences are explored of continuing a heart transplant programme as it was carried out in the period 1985-88. The non-transplant scenario is used to explore the consequences of a political decision to abstain from a heart transplant programme in The Netherlands. The number of donor hearts then equals zero, and costs are calculated on the basis of cost estimates without a transplant programme.

All input sources are obtained from the subsequent sub-studies. Although simulation and estimation are closely related, we will treat them here separately.

Simulations

In the simulation programme, patients who are referred to the transplant centre enter the programme at random times during each year. After entry, the programme simulates a complete patient history, beginning with the duration of screening. In screening, the patient is confronted with four duration distributions: one regarding the duration until death, one regarding the duration until referral to the waiting list, and two regarding duration until a decision that a transplant is definitely or temporarily not recommended. From these, four duration distributions are drawn at random. The shortest duration and the corresponding decision are added to the patient's history. If the shortest duration does not regard survival but, for example, *follow-up*, the process continues. In *follow-up*, the patient is confronted with two possibilities: a return to screening, or death. Again, the shortest duration and the corresponding decision are added to the patient's history. If the duration until a second screening is shortest, that outcome is added to the patient's history, and again the process continues.

With the exception of the duration until transplant, all distributions can be estimated using standard techniques from survival analysis. Excellent textbooks for reference are Kalbfleisch and Prentice [9], Lawless [10], and Cox and Oakes [11].

The probability of being transplanted (or, stated otherwise, the duration until transplant) is affected by the number of donor organs. Therefore no duration distribution can be estimated regarding the time from acceptance on the waiting list until transplantation. Consequently, the model has been divided into two parts: a pre-transplant part, and a post-waiting list part. In the pre-transplant part, which is presented schematically in Figure 2, patient histories are simulated disregarding the possibility of a transplant. This means that all patients referred to the waiting list actually die awaiting transplant.

At the end of the first part, it is known, for each point in time, which patients are on the waiting list. In the second part, which is presented schematically in Figure 3, donor hearts become available at random times during each year.

For each donor, it is checked whether there is any patient on the waiting list. If there are suitable candidates, the donor heart is randomly assigned to one of them. The date of death, which was simulated in the first part of the programme, is set aside, and the patient's history is completed by a new duration: from transplant to death.

At the point of assigning the donor heart to one of the waiting patients, account is taken of one matching criterion. Before entering the programme, each patient and each donor is given a specific blood group which is drawn at random (based on an estimate of the distribution of blood groups in the Dutch population). A transplant is only possible if donor and recipient have compatible blood groups. Account is also taken of the priority rules regarding blood groups, applied when more patients are waiting with compatible blood groups.

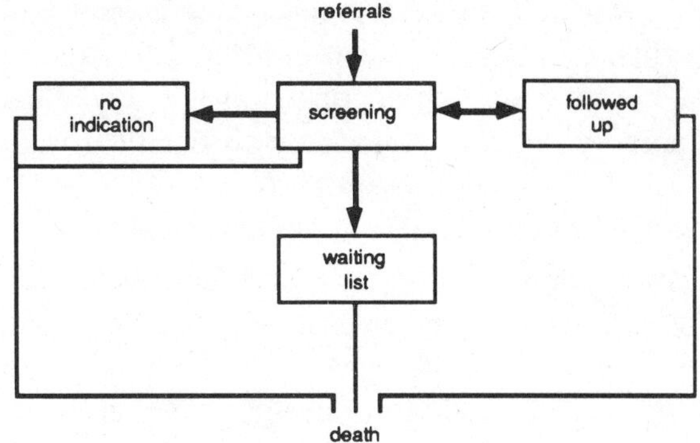

Fig. 2. The Pre-transplant - programme

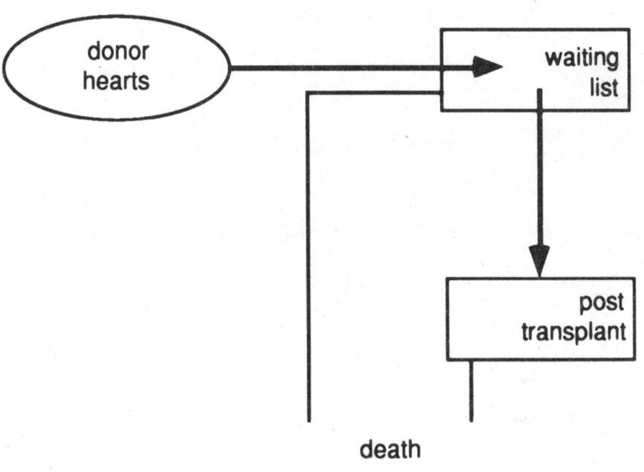

Fig. 3. Post-waiting list programme

Estimation

The numbers of patients referred to the transplant centres were estimated on the basis of the numbers of registered deaths in ICD categories, corrected by selection factors based on expert opinion. The basic estimate for the number referred is 274 patients per year. It was assumed that this number would be reached in 1991, after a linear growth of the number of referrals.

Regarding the number of heart donors, a linear growth was assumed, from 47 in 1987 to 82 in 1994, and so on. The number 82 was estimated on the basis of the yearly number of kidney donors, multiplied by a selection factor which reflects the proportion of multi-organ donors.

Duration of a treatment stage, until death or until some decision is made, is represented by a random variable. In screening, there are four random variables for which the distribution has to be estimated. When a transplant is temporarily not recommended, two durations are of importance. Regarding the waiting list and the post-transplant stage, survival has to be estimated.

Different durations within a treatment stage are analyzed using competing risk models [12]. Related techniques based on survival analysis may also be used. Regarding screening, for example, standard non-parametric tests were used to test for differences between groups, resulting in a distinction between first, second, and third screening. Furthermore, Cox regression was applied to identify trends, showing that a decreasing number of patients were referred with no indication for a heart transplant. This was taken into account by using the estimate for 1 January 1988. On average, 55% of all referred patients are placed on the waiting list, and 38% of these are so placed after a first screening. Twelve percent of referred patients die during screening, and all other patients die while in a treatment stage where there is no indication for transplantation.

Using micro-simulation, heterogeneity within groups can be taken into account. Regarding survival on the waiting list, data on 20 medical variables, including cardiac output and ejection-fraction, were obtained from 137 patients: 53 who had been accepted for transplant, 41 who had definitely no indication, and 43 who had been declared *too healthy*. Cox regression was applied, but *none* of these 20 medical variables showed significant (at the 95% level) effects on survival. Knowing that cardiologists have some implicit appreciation of survival probabilities, the hypothesis was formulated that survival on the waiting list is worse for those patients who are screened in a relatively short period of time, reflecting a sense of urgency. This hypothesis was confirmed by a negative (at the 95% level) coefficient applying Cox regression, with the logarithm of duration of screening as an explanatory variable. (Expert opinion tells us that this *fingerspitzengefühl* is based on the dynamics of some medical variables. This means that not only should values be taken into account, but also first and second order derivates. Therefore longitudinal data would be necessary.) This result was taken into account in further analysis for estimating parametric models. Of these, the exponential model with duration of screening as an explanatory variable, was accepted as the best model. One-year survival was estimated to be 32%, and mean expected survival was estimated to be slightly more than one year (i.e. 400 days).

Technically, this result was taken into account by adding the duration of screening to the patient's history, and by simulating survival on the waiting list using results from the proportional hazards model.

The longest follow-up after transplant was 1 287 days. Because of the absence of reliable sources, survival estimates exceeding 1 287 days have been obtained by extrapolation. Dutch male survival tables were used for this purpose, and it was assumed that survival after the second year after transplantation would be identical to the survival probabilities of the average 69-year-old Dutch male.

The age of 69 years was chosen because of the similarity between survival probabilities at this age and those estimated parametrically for the second and third year after transplantation. Different parametric models were evaluated, and the Pareto model was accepted as the best descriptive model for survival in the first three years after transplantation. Based on these assumptions, the expected survival after transplantation was estimated to be 11.9 years. Ten-year survival was estimated to be 52%, which matches estimates from major transplant centres.

Linking Costs and Effects

The primary results from the micro-simulation programme are patient histories. Cost and effects are calculated subsequently. Effects in terms of life-years are calculated by summing up all durations. Costs and quality-adjusted life-years are calculated by relating the patient histories to the estimates of costs and quality of life.

The relation between the costs and duration of a treatment stage is of importance if assumptions are made that affect the average duration of a treatment stage. In the heart transplant programme, the average duration is affected by two treatment stages: duration on the waiting list, and duration after transplant. The average duration on the waiting list is affected by the interaction of the future number of donor organs and the future number of patients on the waiting list. The average survival after transplant differed from the observed average survival because no long-term data were available. It is assumed that the average duration of screening will not change in the future. One may therefore calculate average costs per patient, and disregard the relation between costs and duration.

In the heart transplant study, data on costs were available for each point of time. On the basis of these data, the relation between duration of a treatment stage and total costs could be analyzed. Thus costs per day after entry into a treatment stage were estimated by summing up the costs per day after entry, divided by the number of patients about whom data were available on that day. Subsequently, an estimate of the cumulative cost curve was obtained by summing up the chronological estimates of costs per day. This method, which was named the Sum-Limit method, through analogy with the Product-Limit method in survival analysis, has some distinct advantages. First, no assumptions have to be made about the relation between costs and duration: the method is non-parametric. Second, sudden increases are identified, for example due to yearly follow-up costs, and bias due to incomplete follow-up is minimized. Third, as in linear regression, the sum of the residuals equals zero. (This means that, if duration per patient is taken into account, observed average costs per patient equal estimated costs per patient.)

The result of the Sum-Limit method is a stepwise non-decreasing function. Costs are estimated as the result of a stochastic process, in which the probability of generating costs depends on the time from entry into a treatment stage. It should be noted, however, that if the length of stay in some treatment stage depends on certain therapeutic actions to be taken, the Sum-Limit method leads to biased estimates.

Thus costs were analyzed per treatment stage. Costs during screening ranged between fl. 4 500 (Dutch guilders) for patients with definitely no indication, and fl. 12 000 for patients referred to the waiting list. Costs on the waiting list were estimated, taking into account length of stay. With transplant, programme costs were estimated at fl. 64 000 per year, and without transplant, at fl 53 000. Costs were estimated at fl. 141 000 during the first year after transplantation, and in later years at about fl. 37 000 a year. All these results can be linked directly to each patient's history.

An identical methodology may be applied concerning quality of life. In the heart transplant study, a very simple procedure was followed. Life-years before transplant were multiplied by a factor of 0.225, and life-years after transplant by a factor of 0.7. This estimate of the improvement in quality of life after transplant was based mainly on computer-assisted interviews. In addition, use was made of a model which was developed for translating health states into values on a zero-to-one scale. On the basis of this model, quality of life before transplant was estimated to lie within the range of 0.15-0.30. Quality of life after transplant was estimated to lie within the range of 0.55-0.85 [3].

Some Results

The results presented here are the averages of one hundred simulation runs. Table 1 shows the numbers of patients entering the waiting list, the number of donor hearts, and the number of transplants. Table 2 shows the numbers of patients alive at given years after being placed on the waiting list, with and without a transplant programme. The annual number of transplants, and the number of donor hearts, are expected to stabilize in 1994, with 80 transplants performed in that year. It appears that the number of patients who will be alive after transplant will continue to rise during this century. The difference between the number of patients alive with and without transplant will also continue to increase. The number of patients alive at the beginning of the next century, who would have been dead without a transplant programme, is predicted to be 534.

Table 3 presents the yearly costs with a transplant programme per treatment stage. The post-transplant costs include the costs of transplantation. In 1988, the cost of operation was 11,5% of post-transplant costs. In 1999, it will be less than 5%, and more than 95% of post-transplant costs will be related to treatment after operation.

Table 4 shows estimates of costs in the non-transplant programme per treatment stage. Costs due to treatment of transplanted patients will account for more than 70% of total programme costs. This proportion is increasing. It is predicted that total yearly costs will not exceed 42 million guilders. Costs that would have occurred without a transplant programme increase less steeply than those with a transplant programme. The latter is expected to be around 10 million guilders in 1999. Hence, while it is predicted that, in 1999, there will be more than 500 patients alive as a result of a heart transplant, the estimated *net* cost is 31 million guilders.

Table 1. Donor hearts and patients after placement on the waiting list: The Netherlands 1988-1999

Year	Donor hearts	Patients placed on the waiting list	Transplants
1988	52	89	48
1992	72	145	70
1996	82	147	80
1999	82	149	80

Table 2. Patients alive at given years, with and without a transplant programme

Year	With transplant programme	Without transplant programme
1988	127	48
1992	356	131
1996	564	152
1999	693	159

Discussion

The Dutch heart transplant programme has been modelled as a stochastic compartment model, using the micro-simulation technique. The primary reason for

Table 3. The Dutch transplant programme: annual costs 1988-1999 (fl. 1 000)

Year	Screening	Second/third screening	Waiting list	Post-transplant	Programme costs	Total
1988	1 991	445	1 528	7 902	1 214	13 080
1992	3 024	877	4 221	17 318	1 791	27 231
1996	3 012	928	4 102	26 259	2 028	36 329
1999	3 015	958	4 113	31 220	2 023	41 329

Table 4. The Dutch transplant programme: yearly costs without a transplant programme 1988-1999 (fl. 1 000)

Year	First screening	Second/third screening	Waiting list	Total
1988	859	182	1 602	2 634
1992	1 302	358	6 579	8 239
1996	1 297	379	7 924	9 600
1999	1 298	391	8 237	9 962

this choice was its ability to take account of the interaction between survival, numbers of patients, and a limited number of donor organs. In this respect it has proved successful.

In addition, micro-simulation has the advantage that it fits perfectly with standard techniques which have been developed to estimate duration distributions. Results from these techniques can be applied directly to the simulation programme. Moreover, results from more advanced techniques, such as estimates which take account of unobserved heterogeneity, or of local independence, may be implemented directly. The effect of lags and time-dependent explanatory variables may also be included.

Forecasting cost and effects was also shown to be possible. Direct links can be made between the simulated patient histories, and estimates of costs and quality of life per treatment stage. Costs and effects of different scenarios can be estimated.

Disadvantages of micro-simulation are related to computer time and computer space. Heart transplantation concerns only about 300 patients a year. One hundred simulation runs take about 3 hours on an IBM personal computer. For calculations at the population level, therefore, more power is needed, otherwise whole generations may have died before their prognoses have been calculated.

References

1. van Hout BA, Habbema JDF, Bonsel GJ (1988) Costs and effects of heart transplantation. Report 5: Prognoses of heart transplantations. Erasmus University, Rotterdam, p 74
2. van Hout BA, Idele M, de Charro FT (1988) Costs and effects of heart transplantation. Report 6: The costs of heart transplantation. Erasmus University, Rotterdam, p 55
3. Bonsel GJ, Boterblom A, Bot ML, van't Veer F (1988) Costs and effects of heart transplantation. Report 2: Quality of life. Erasmus University, Rotterdam, p 272
4. de Charro FTH, Bonsel GJ, Bot ML (1989) Costs and effects of heart transplantation. Report 7: The supply of donor organs. Erasmus University, Rotterdam, p 25
5. Bot M, Bonsel GJ, van't Veer F (1988) Costs and effects of heart transplantation. Report 8: The need for heart transplantation. Erasmus University, Rotterdam, p 94
6. van Hout BA, Habbema JDF (1988) Costs and effects of heart transplantation. Report 4: Scenarios of the Dutch heart transplant programme. Erasmus University, Rotterdam, p 96
7. Manton KG, Stallard E (1988) Chronic Disease Modelling. Oxford University Press, New York, p 279
8. Davies H, Davies R (1987) A simulation model for planning services for renal patients in Europe. Journal of the operational research society 38:693-700
9. Kalbfleisch JD, Prentice RL (1980) The statistical analysis of failure time data. Wiley, New York, p 321
10. Lawless JF (1982) Statistical models and methods for lifetime data. Wiley, New York, p 537
11. Cox DR, Oakes D (1984) Analysis of survival data. Chappman and Hall, Cambridge, p 201
12. David HA, Moeschberger ML (1978) The theory of competing risks. Griffin's Statistical Monographs and Courses no. 39 , Griffin, London, p 103

Regional Variation in Risk Factor Distributions and National CHD Mortality in Europe - with a View Towards Disease Modelling

W. Morgenstern on behalf of the WHO ERICA Research Group
(based on a presentation at the 2nd World Conference on Preventive Cardiology, Washington DC, 1989)

This paper deals with one of the common methodological problems in disease modelling: the link between risk factors of diseases and morbidity or mortality from diseases on the one hand and the usual lack of *optimal* data for this link on the other hand. It will be demonstrated by exploratory data analysis that it is possible to establish a link between local risk factor distributions and national mortality rates. The repercussions of this on disease modelling are obvious.

Methods

The data analyzed in this paper come from two different sources: national mortality statistics provided by the World Health Organization (WHO), and risk factor distributions of sample surveys provided by the WHO ERICA (European Risk and Incidence, a Coordinated Analysis) Research Group. The ERICA Project is a study of coronary heart disease (CHD), which collected epidemiological survey data from the European region. It is a retrospective analysis of surveys performed in the 1970's. Risk factor distributions from 35 surveys in 17 European countries have been published [1].

The basic question for the present investigation was to determine whether risk factor distributions in local geographical areas can provide reasonable estimates of national CHD mortality rates. At the first stage of our analysis, we chose linear regression models in which the national CHD mortality rate is used as the dependent variable and estimates of mortality – computed from local risk factor distributions – are used as independent variables.

The ERICA-surveys are used for estimating national CHD mortality rates. This has been done by means of coefficients of multiple logistic functions (MLF) for the parameters age, cholesterol, systolic blood pressure, body mass index and cigarette smoking. The coefficients, based on the iterative solution of the logistic regression of Walker and Duncan [2], were calculated in the ERICA-Project. Results of these computations were published in detail by the ERICA Research Group [3]. So far, ERICA was mainly concerned with males, aged 40-59 years. Therefore, our analysis is restricted to this gender and to these age-groups.

The MLFs in ERICA are derived from 12 studies which have a minimum of five-year mortality follow-up (comprising approx. 21.000 individuals). Coefficients are elaborated by various geographical groupings of the studies. These coefficients are then applied to the risk factor distributions of 28 ERICA-studies including those 16 with no mortality follow-up. Out of the 35 ERICA studies seven are excluded (five studies of the USSR for which national mortality statistics are not available and two studies which included only single-year age classes). National cause-specific mortality is available for five-year age-groups. We apply the MLFs separately to the following age-groups: 40-44 years, 45-49 years, 50-54 years, and 55-59 years. Estimated standardized death rates (SDR) are then calculated for each survey population on the basis of those MLFs. These estimates refer to a five-year period based on the pattern of the initial risk factors in the specific surveys. In order to calculate the national mortality rates for the same period of time, the respective age-specific national mortality rates for the survey-year and for the fifth year following the survey are added, divided by 2 and multiplied by five. The rate is then expressed as SDR (the European standard population serves as a reference population [4]).

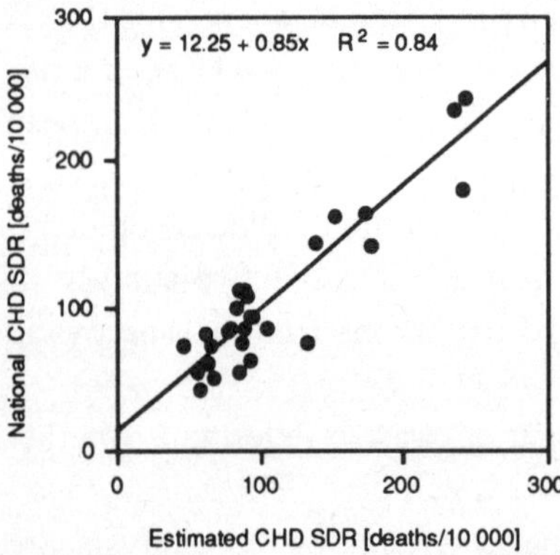

Fig. 1. National CHD standardized deaths rates (SDR) and MLF estimates of CHD SDR in local survey populations (28 studies). MLFs were derived from pools of four different European regions

Results

Coefficients of MLF derived from various, regional geographical groupings of the studies are used in the evaluation. The best results are obtained by those estimates based on MLF coefficients which were derived from four different pools, each representing four different European regions. The definition of the four geographical regions (North, South, West and East Europe) is given in [1]. For each of the 28 surveys the estimates have been calculated according to the specific European region to which the survey belongs, i.e. according to the region's specific MLF. The graph of the regression is given in Figure 1. As can be seen, the overall correspondence is fairly good. Most of the points are located close to the regression line. The R^2 shows that 84% of the variation observed in national CHD SDRs is explained by estimates derived from these MLF-coefficients. The slope (0.85) and the intercept (12.25) result in an overestimation of national CHD SDRs. The regression indicates, however, that for males aged 40-59 years the relation between national CHD mortality and local risk factor distributions is good. This is the case when regional coefficients are used.

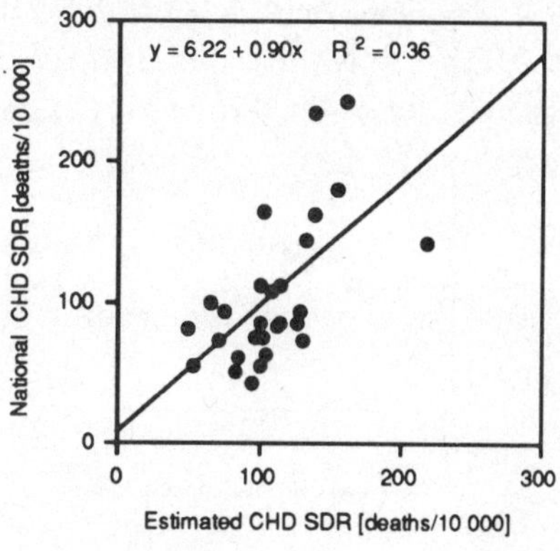

Fig. 2. National CHD standardized deaths rates (SDR) and MLF estimates of CHD SDR in local survey populations (28 studies). MLFs were derived from one pool for the whole of Europe

Next, we compare this result with another one which we achieved by applying a uniform MLF for the whole of Europe, i.e. a MLF deriving from one pool comprising all 12 studies with mortality follow-up. This regression is given in Figure 2. Compared with the regression described above, the result is rather poor. Only 36% of the overall variation observed in national CHD SDRs is explained. Risk factor distributions of males of that age (as well as CHD mortality) show larger variation in the European region in the 1970's [1]. The application of a single MLF seems to fail in assessing this variation. This may lead to an outcome similar to that described for instance by Menotti et al. [5], which indicated that the application of risk functions from one cultural entity to another may result in poor predictions.

When we divided Europe into two regions and combined North and West Europe with its high risk factor prevalences in the 1970's and East and South Europe with its lower prevalences [1], we found a stronger relation between national CHD SDRs and MLF-estimates (the results are not given here), but still less strong than the relation described in Figure 1.

Next, we investigated whether the strong relation observed between national CHD SDR and MLF-estimates achieved by applying regional MLFs, is caused by a real relation between risk factor distributions in local areas and national CHD mortality or by the mechanism of the MLF itself as a logistic regression which, of course, predicts exactly the mortality of the population from which it is derived.

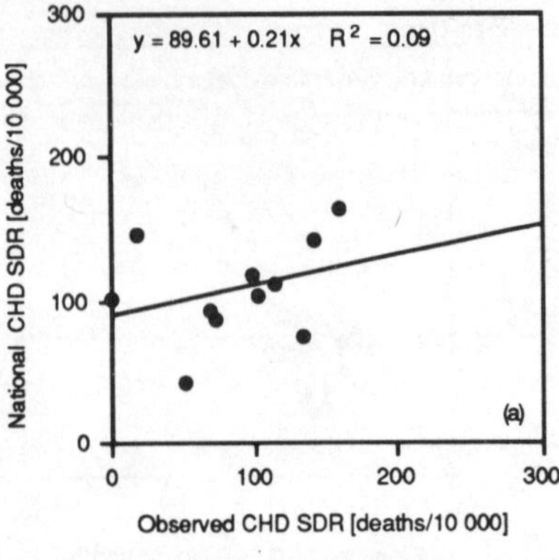

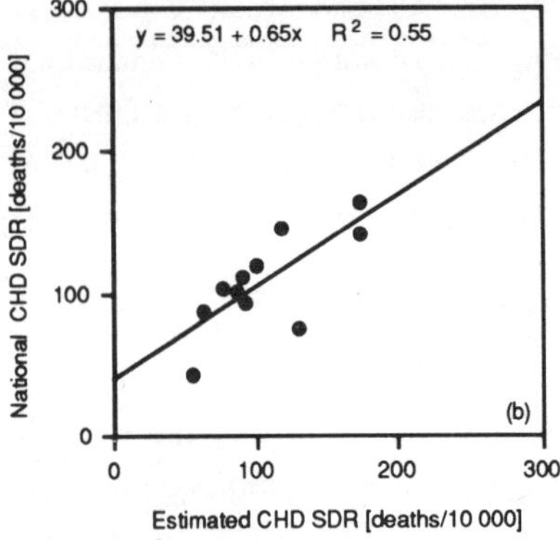

Fig. 3. National CHD standardized deaths rates (SDR) and (a) observed CHD SDR (b) MLF estimates of CHD SDR in local survey populations (11 studies with follow-up). MLFs were derived from pools of four different European regions

For this investigation we used only 11 of the 12 surveys having a mortality follow-up from which the regional MLFs are derived (one of the 12 surveys was excluded because national statistics were not available). First, we investigated the relation of the true CHD mortality observed in the survey populations and the national mortality. The result of this regression is shown in Figure 3 (a). Only 9% of the overall variation in the national CHD SDR was explained by the mortality observed in local areas. This outcome is reflected in the estimate of the error term (89.51). When applying the four regional MLFs to the risk factor distribution in these surveys, we obtain a distinctly better result, as shown in Figure 3(b) (Note, that the survey data have been pooled to evaluate the regional MLFs). Here, 55% of the variation is explained and the estimate of the error term is 39.51. This may indicate that the interaction between risk factor and CHD mortality given by the four regional MLFs can be used to estimate national mortality from CHD risk factor distributions. Furthermore, the poor prediction of national CHD mortality on the basis of mortality rates observed in small local areas on the one hand and the better prediction on the basis of MLF-estimates derived from pooled data from such small surveys in a larger European region on the other hand, may indicate that local risk factor distributions do not sufficiently reflect the variation in larger regions. In Table 1 the four linear regression models described here are summarized.

Discussion

The main goal of disease modelling in larger populations is to support health policy planning. For the time being the modelling will provide the possibility of

Tab. 1. Linear regression models. National CHD standardized deaths rates (SDR) as dependent variable. Estimated CHD SDR in local survey populations as independent variable. Model I is based on MLFs from pools of four different European Regions (28 studies). Model II is based on MLFs from one pool for the whole of Europe (28 studies). Model III is based on observed CHD SDR in survey populations of 11 studies with follow-up. Model IV is based on MLFs from pools of four different European regions (11 studies with follow-up)

	Model I		Model II		Model III		Model IV	
Model		$p < 0.001$		$p < 0.001$		$p = 0.364$		$p < 0.01$
Intercept	12.246	$p = 0.179$	6.217	$p = 0.818$	89.562	$p < 0.01$	39.510	$p = 0.105$
Estimated CHD SDR	0.849	$p < 0.001$	0.903	$p < 0.01$	0.207	$p = 0.364$	0.646	$p < 0.01$
R^2	0.841		0.364		0.092		0.548	

simulations, i.e. it will allow playing with scenarios under different assumptions, rather than providing a deterministic, quantitatively exact projection. In this kind of modelling, simulations of changes in mortality attributable to changes in risk factors play an important part, e.g. in planning national prevention campaigns, mass screenings etc. Prerequisites for this sort of modelling are predictive factors which can be expressed mathematically for the modelling purposes. With respect to CHD, it is well-known that such relations exist in general for a number of risk factors. The relations found seem to be reliable. At least for a specific gender and age-group (males, 40-59 years), we demonstrate that national CHD mortality rates can be linked to CHD risk factor distributions observed in local areas. Logistic regression appears to be a useful tool for expressing functional relationships.

The MLFs, which are used and evaluated in the ERICA-Project, yield good results and thus seem to be appropriate for modelling-purposes. However, it should be kept in mind that ERICA is a retrospective analysis of studies conducted in the 1970's. Since that time considerable changes have been taking place in the European regions, for instance, a pronounced decrease of CHD mortality in the North and West region (e.g. Finland) and on the other hand a dramatic increase in Eastern countries (e.g. Hungary). There are some indicators (Gyarfas and Morgenstern, unpublished paper) that these changes are also reflected by changes in risk factors. At present the ERICA-MLFs are the only ones which cover larger regions in Europe.

In the linear regression models national CHD mortality during a five-year interval was determined by calculating the average mortality rate reported for the years of the interval. It is of course evident, that these mean values do not represent exact figures since the increase of mortality in these cohorts will be exponential instead of linear, even in a five-year period. This error is likely to be relatively constant, however, and is not expected to have substantial effects on the regression model.

We obtained promising results when we applied different MLFs derived from ERICA data. The best result we attained was based on MLFs which were separately established for the North, East, South and West European regions. A poor result was achieved by using a single MLF for the whole of Europe. From this we conclude that a *unique* European MLF does not assess the variation due to different traditions and cultures. Thus the predictive power of the logistic regression is low with respect to the estimation of national CHD mortality based on local risk factor distributions. On the other hand, we demonstrate that true CHD mortality rates observed in smaller local areas are even less useful for predicting national mortality rates. Obviously one fails to assess variation here as well.

From the results described here one may conclude that 1) the *regionality* of a disease has to be assessed, i.e. has to be expressed functionally and 2) that in attempting this, generalization, as well as specification, may fail in their extremes. Therefore modelling should be performed adaptively.

Finally, it should be stressed once more that the paper deals only with the question of whether a link between local risk factor distributions and national CHD mortality seems to be reasonable.

References

1. ERICA Research Group (1988) The CHD Risk-map of Europe. The 1st report of the WHO-ERICA Project. Eur Heart J 9 Suppl 1: 1-36
2. Walker SH, Duncan DB (1967) Estimation of the probability of an event as a function of several independent variables. Biometrika 54: 167-179
3. ERICA Research Group (1991) Prediction of coronary heart disease in Europe. The 2nd report of the WHO-ERICA Project. Eur Heart J 12: 291-297
4. International Agency for Research on Cancer (1976) Cancer Incidence in Five Continents. IARC Scientific Publ 15: 456
5. Menotti A, Capocaccia R, Farchi G (1982) Stima dell' incidenza di cardiopatia coronarica in una popolazione impiegando la funzione di rischio di un'altra. Rev Lat Cardiol 3: 461-466

Printing: Weihert-Druck GmbH, Darmstadt
Binding: Buchbinderei Schäffer, Grünstadt